Your Ultimate Surgery Success Guide

Practical Strategies to Guide You Step-by-Step from Surgery Stress to Surgery Success

ELLE PENDRICK

Praise for *Your Ultimate Surgery Success Guide*

"This package is a unique and really valuable practical resource for people undergoing open heart surgery."

- A/Professor Rachael Cordina, Cardiologist

"I have no doubt that this will be very helpful for people who find themselves in Elle's position or even for parents who are supervising the management of their children."

- Dr Steven Cooper, Paediatric Cardiologist

"I have found this comprehensive guide filled with wisdom and compassion – a great guide not only for people going through surgery but a helpful read for their support team as well."

- Maureen Germein, Mental Health Social Worker

"Elle's book is a comprehensive guide that ensures every beat is accounted for. From pre-surgery considerations to surgery day and post-surgery care, Elle has presented all the information into easily digestible sections with actionable steps and tips before the big day."

- Jenna Cantamessa, Partner of Open Heart Surgery Survivor

"This is a great book! I learned some fantastic strategies, tips and tricks that are making my surgery journey far more manageable. Highly Recommend!"

- Lloyd Johnson, Preparing for Open Heart Surgery

"This book was a lifesaver. I couldn't have gotten through surgery, prepared my family, and been a more sane and zen person doing it. Thank you, thank you, thank you!!!"

- Nova Inkpen, Preparing for Open Heart Surgery

Creator: Pendrick, Elle

Title: Your Ultimate Surgery Success Guide: Practical Strategies to Guide You Step-by-Step from Surgery Stress to Surgery Success

ISBN: 9798336397048 (Hardback) | ISBN: 9798335249164 (Paperback)

Disclaimer
The information provided in this book is designed to be general in nature, to provide a strong foundation for all. However, everybody's situation and goals are unique so I cannot guarantee that your desired outcome will be met. It is not intended to provide specific guidance for particular circumstances and it should not be relied on as the basis for any decision to take action or not take action on any matter which it covers. The information provided is not a substitute for independent professional legal, regulatory, business, or financial advice and any reliance on this information is at your sole risk. I am not a financial advisor or lawyer. You must consider whether or not the information is appropriate to your needs. I strongly recommend that you obtain independent professional advice before making any decisions or taking steps towards reliance on this information. The information provided is also not a substitute for independent professional health or medical advice. Participation in this book, action plan and community group is voluntary and is always at your sole risk. To the maximum extent permitted by law, the author disclaims all responsibility and liability to any person, arising directly or indirectly from any person taking or not taking action based on the information in this publication. For full terms and conditions, see here: https://www.adultingwell.au/ebook-course-T&C

The author is not affiliated with and does not endorse any of the corporate entities mentioned in or involved in the distribution of this work, or any third party entities whose trademarks and logos may appear in this work.

"This book is dedicated to all past, present, and future surgery survivors whose strength and resilience inspire us all. May these pages be a source of companionship, practicality, and reassurance."

By Elle Pendrick, Founder of Adulting Well

Your Ultimate Surgery Success Guide

includes...

- **15 Budget Strategies** to Save You Money and Get Every Cent You're Entitled To (and not a cent less)
- **9 Workplace Tactics** to Negotiate with Your Boss, Manage Your Workplace, and Keep Your Career
- **8 Tips for Choosing the Right Hospital for Surgery**
- **8 Scripts** with Exactly What to Say to Your Boss, Insurance, and Loved Ones
- **12 Questions to Ask Your Surgeon Right Now**
- **10 Mindset Hacks** Guaranteed to Ease the Pressure
- **7 Coms Strategies** to Help Your Loved Ones Cope
- **19 People You Need** and How to Find Them
- **13 Must-Have Items for Your Hospital Bag**
- **7 Tried-and-Tested Ways to Cope in Hospital**
- **17 Questions to Ask Before You Leave Hospital**
- **15 Tech Hacks** that Will Make Your Life Easier
- **11 Steps for Your Road to Recovery**
- **37 Practical Action Steps** to Achieve Your Goals
- **44 Bonus Tips** to Give You the Extra Edge
- **60 Personal Quotes** to Inspire and Motivate You
- **FREE Action Plan** So You Can Personalise Every Step
- **FREE Online Support Group Access** to Have All Your Questions Answered and Be Around People Like You
- **And Much More!**

Table of Contents

PART 3 - IN HOSPITAL

PART 4 - RECOVERY

PART 5 - END NOTES

PART 1

INTRODUCTION

CHAPTER 01

My Story

Hello!

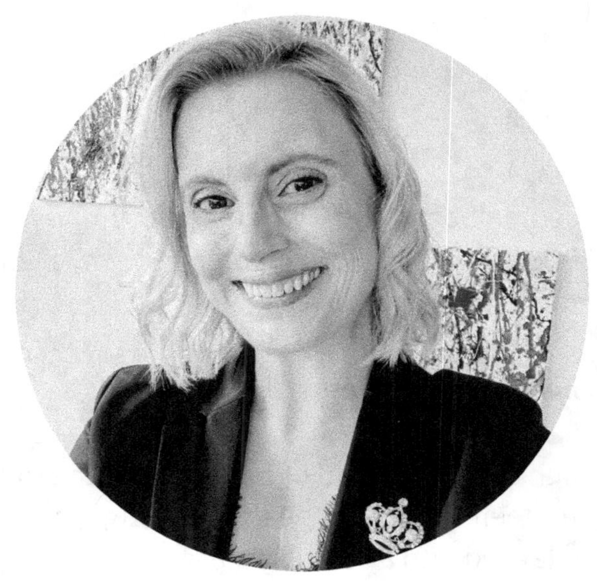

I'm your guide, Elle, a 5-time open-heart surgery survivor.

I know first-hand that surgery impacts every part of your life, from your mindset to budgeting and navigating the workplace. It leaves no stone unturned.

That's why I've written this book to cover it all. Here, you'll find practical strategies to guide you step-by-step from Surgery Stress to Surgery Success.

You're not alone - I've been right where you are. You've got this, and I've got you!

Elle Pendrick

Adultingwell.au
hello@adultingwell.au

My Story

I couldn't believe it. I was utterly numb and shell shocked. It was 2016 and I was barely holding onto my phone while staring at an email.

I needed my fifth open heart surgery.

Then came the flood of memories of the four other surgeries, the umpteen catheters, the hospital stays, and the recovery. I collapsed into a sobbing mess.

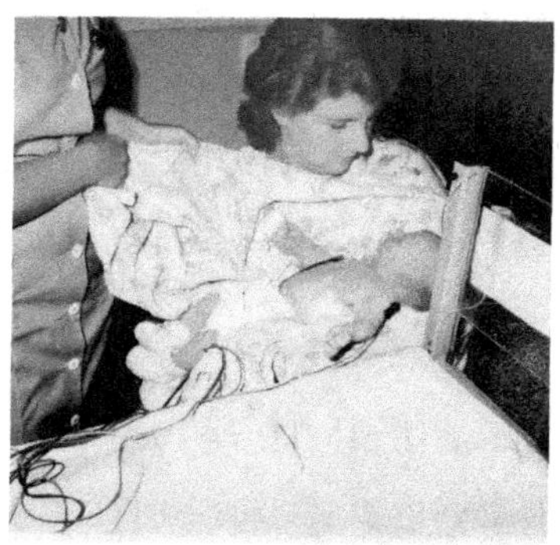

1983 - 6 Days Old - 3 Days After My First Open Heart Surgery

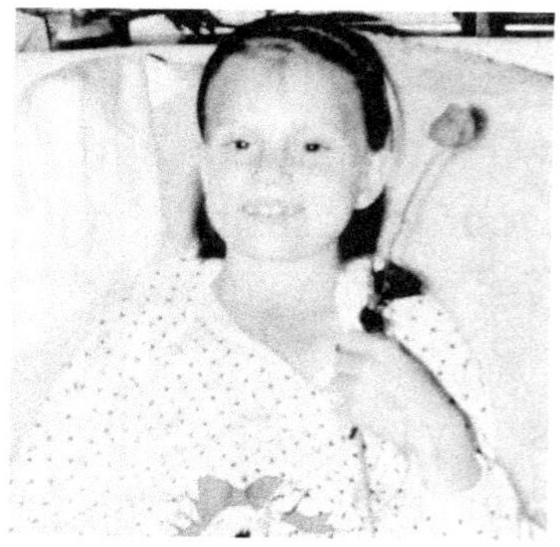

1989 - 6 Years Old - 5 Days After My Second Open Heart Surgery

Logically, I knew I needed the surgery to stay alive and have any kind of life. But I couldn't bear the thought of what I'd have to go through to get there, yet again.

I remembered all too vividly the long, dark days waiting for the surgery, where I'd go over and over things. That led to sleepless nights. I was lost for words when trying to tell my loved ones the news. I remember being overwhelmed trying to figure out how I was going to pay my bills. Fumbling my way through sorting my leave and uni, not knowing what I was even entitled to.

I remembered the dry and boring information from the hospital. It was so useless that I threw it in the bin. Waiting in the cold and sterile hospital with its never-ending hallways. I remember waking up after surgery and being disorientated and unable to talk. When I finally could talk, I told my family to 'piss off' because it was too overwhelming.

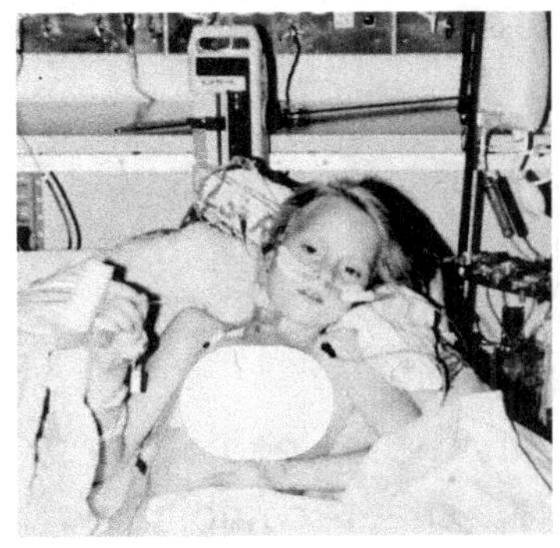

1991 – 8 Years Old – 2 Days After My Third Open Heart Surgery

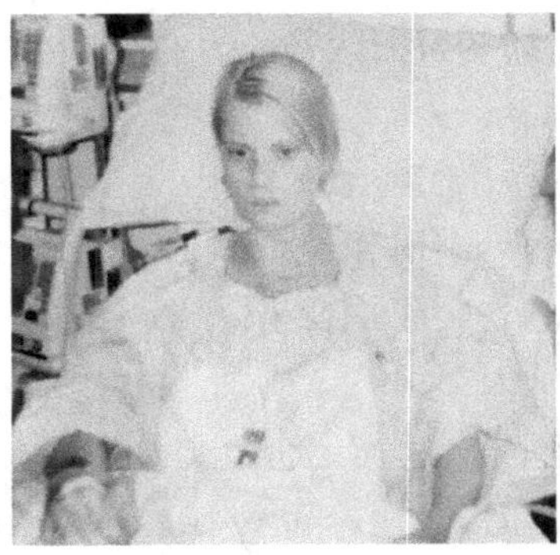

2004 – 21 Years Old – 3 Days After My Fourth Open Heart Surgery

"I remember feeling alone and scared."

The pain and distress continued when I got home and realised we'd forgotten some of the medication I needed. We had to spend hours with doctors and pharmacists sorting it out. Every night, I woke up with dread under the heavy doona, not being sure if I could get myself out of bed. I hated the rubbish rehab plan the hospital sent me home with. I was so confused about when I could and couldn't do things like driving, hanging out washing, and even having sex.

Safe to say, I was overwhelmed and thoroughly terrified. I never wanted another surgery. Ever!

But that wasn't the reality I lived in.

After I really wallowed and swam around in my feelings, I gathered whatever crumbs of courage I had and scoured the internet desperately for a guide, for help, for something—anything —that would give me inspiration and practical ways to tackle this.

I found plenty of dry, boring, personality-less fact sheets filled with stuff I already knew. But I didn't find a single thing that resonated with me.

After days of going around in circles, it finally dawned on me: I already knew way more than all these fact sheets combined!

*"I had already lived it. I had already
survived it. Four times over!"*

This was not my first rodeo! In fact, it wasn't my first, second, third, or even fourth. This was my fifth open heart surgery!

I knew exactly what to expect. I knew all the aspects of my life that this surgery would impact. I knew I'd done it four other times, and my life was better after each one.

So, I dug deep, really deep, and decided to tackle this head-on. I decided to approach this surgery with practicality and purpose. I decided to own the fact that I was having surgery (yet again).

*"I decided to make this my
best surgery ever."*

I made my mindset my number one priority, connecting with a mental health professional who really understood. She helped me handle anxiety and set me up with practical tips. I also found online meditation and hypnosis to ease my worries. Writing my feelings down at night was like venting to a friend.

My family pitched in without a fuss; it wasn't their first rodeo either. But for my husband and me, it was our first. Heartfelt discussions and meal preparation united us, fostering a new level of support.

I made the tough call and put my health first, taking a break from my dream job. After doing my homework and discussing it with the Human Resources department, I confidently negotiated leave. They were so supportive.

My research led to an informed decision about which hospital to go to, while self-made signs to communicate post-op, new pj's, and playlists set the stage for a positive experience.

From a visitor plan to post-surgery meals, I had it all sorted. When I walked into the hospital, I was scared, but ready to face surgery.

When I woke up from surgery, my prep helped me cope better. As soon as I could, I played my favourite songs and let my mind wander with meditation. I turned the noisy hospital into peaceful forests and sunny beaches.

I used those pre-made signs to communicate. I'm proud to say that I didn't tell my family to piss off. That sign still goes unused.

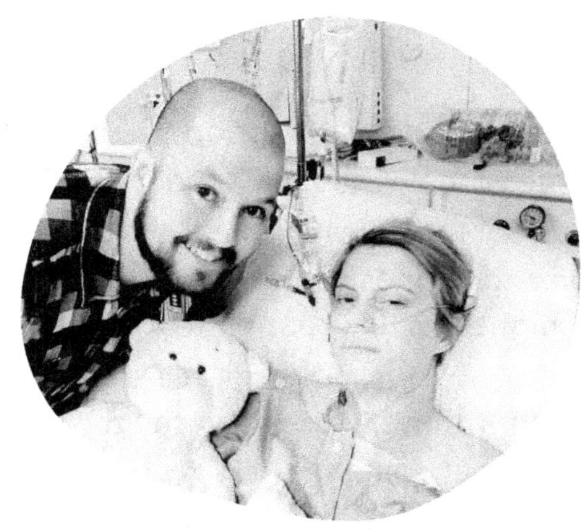

2016 - 33 Years Old - 2 Days After My Fifth Open Heart Surgery with My Husband Adam Buck

Every little victory, like sitting up, having a meal, and even having a poo, was a step toward getting back to my best life.

My care team was awesome. They adapted to my likes and avoided what I didn't like. Even when things didn't go perfectly, I focused on the good stuff.

When it was time to leave, I had my questions ready. They showed me how to get out of bed on my own and told me when I could drive and do chores again. We even tackled the awkward topic of sex.

On the drive home, I made sure I was comfy with pillows, and we had great food and entertainment waiting. We did forget one pain med (oops!), but this time, I knew how to sort it out fast.

Rehab was a game-changer. I had a fantastic physio at the hospital, and once home, I went to full-on rehab classes twice a week for months.

All my planning paid off. Within six months, I was hiking in Hawaii, working back in my dream job, and living my best life!

I had succeeded and had my best surgery ever.

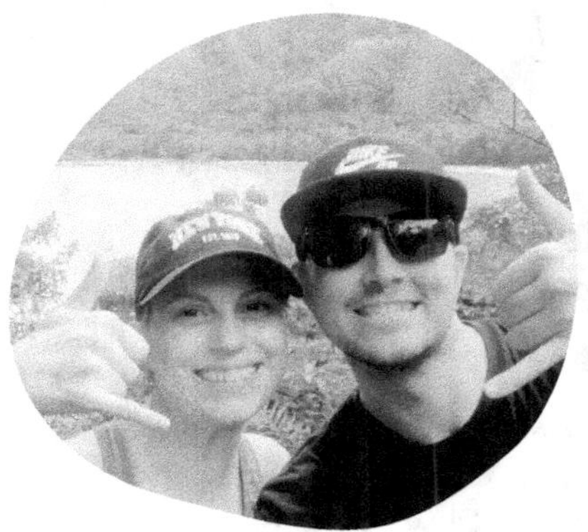

2017 - 33 Years Old - 6 Months After My Fifth Open Heart Surgery with My Husband Adam Buck in Hawaii

"I really wanted to share my story with you because it proved to me that by shifting your mindset, being super practical, and having a little fun along the way, you can do ANYTHING."

If you're facing major surgery and can relate to my story, I've got you. I truly get it. I've been where you are quite a few times. I hear you, I see you, and I feel you.

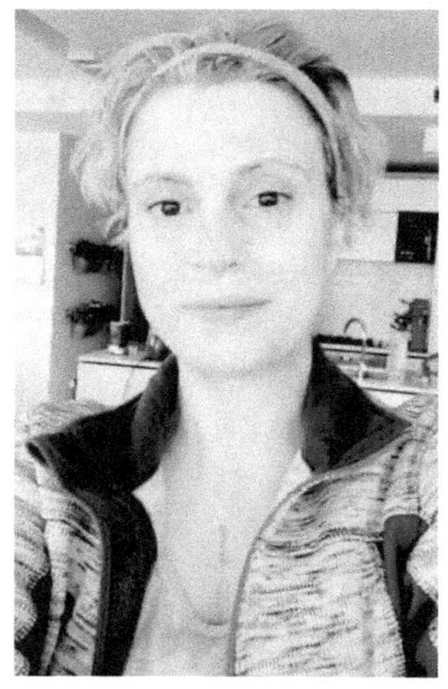

"I'm determined to make sure no one ever has to go through major surgery without a guide."

2016 - 33 Years Old - 3 Months After My Fifth Open Heart Surgery

I was so determined that I wrote the guide myself. My first blog, 'Open Heart Surgery–Tips n Tricks from a Pro,' went viral in 2018 with thousands of views. Hundreds of people reached out to share their stories and how the guide had helped them have their best surgery.

Since then, I've learnt even more and have put together a more in-depth and practical guide, complete with a personalised action plan. Just for you.

In these pages you'll find everything you need for Surgery Success. Practicality will be your superpower and laughter will be your best medicine.

With this book, you'll have everything you need to guide you to achieving the mindset you want, sorting money and work, making tough decisions, preparing for each step, and celebrating every win through hospital and recovery.

Now, get in the ring!

"You've got this, and
I've got you."

CHAPTER 02

How to Use the Book

Using the Book

WHO IS THE BOOK FOR?

EVERYONE! This book is dedicated to people going through surgery. However, it's also for their carers, colleagues, healthcare professionals, hospital staff, charities, financial institutions, bureaucrats and anyone else who is touched by someone going through major surgery.

This is for you if **you're going in for major surgery**, like open heart surgery, a transplant, cancer removal, joint replacement, or any other type of major surgery. If you've already had your surgery or it's just days away, that's okay. Take from the book what you need right now and come back to it as a resource when you need it.

If you're **caring for someone** going through major surgery, this book will help you navigate everything and see things from their perspective. Sometimes, people having major surgery may not be well enough to do all the practical stuff, so you can use this to help them or do it for them.

If you're a **health professional, hospital staff member, charity worker, bureaucrat, boss, or colleague,** the book will give you a unique perspective of what someone is contending with for their major surgery. It will help you provide better service and be more compassionate, as you'll understand the full scope of what they are facing. It's not just about the surgical procedure!

NAVIGATING THE BOOK

This book was written so you can skip around and pick n' choose the chapters that interest you the most... but surgery impacts your whole life, so to ace it, you should read it all.

You might come across some parts that make you feel a bit uncomfortable. That's okay and perfectly normal. You can skip that chunk and come back to it when you're ready. Don't put down the whole book because of one part, there is loads of other useful information in here.

YOUR PERSPECTIVE

As a white woman from a middle-class family in regional Australia, I probably haven't had the same life experiences as you. That's why I've done a lot of homework and chatted to loads of people to try and prep you for experiences that I might not have had, but you might.

I'm also not a professional in any of the areas in this book, unless you count five open heart surgeries and 40 years of living with chronic illness! Take away from it what you need for your situation. Do your own homework!

AUSSIE PERSPECTIVE

The book has been entirely written from an Aussie perspective. From laws to healthcare systems, it's all for Aussies. But it can absolutely still be handy to people outside the great land of Oz. The foundations are the same, particularly around mindset.

Resource Library

Check out these resources specially designed to help you along your surgery success journey.

ACTION PLAN - FREE

Your Action Plan is your personalised roadmap, carefully crafted to help you navigate your surgery journey like a pro. From practical checklists for packing your hospital bag to sorting your budget, this plan has it all!

Markers throughout the book say 'Action Step,' showing you when to whip out your Action Plan to make your own notes, plans, and strategies. Take it everywhere with you. Make notes and be messy.

SCAN THE QR CODE TO ACCESS GET YOUR FREE PLAN

https://www.adultingwell.au/Action-Plan-YUSSG

SURGERY SQUAD - FREE

Are you ready for the ultimate cheer squad while conquering your surgery journey like a boss? Say hello to the 'Adulting Well – Surgery Squad'.

It's a virtual forum where we spill the tea, laugh, cry, and cheer each other on through this wild ride together! Need some candid advice on hospital hacks? We gotchu! Wanna share your packing list? We're all ears! Feeling nervous but can't admit it to your nearest and dearest? No worries, we get it!

Inside the Adulting Well – Surgery Squad, we're all about creating a judgment-free zone where you can be your authentic self. Whether you're pumped to ace this journey or just need a virtual shoulder to lean on, we've got you covered!

SCAN THE QR CODE TO ACCESS THE SURGERY SQUAD

Facebook - Adulting Well Surgery Squad

BLOGS & EMAILS - FREE

Get a regular dose of inspiration, practical tips, and heartfelt support right to your inbox with the Adulting Well blogs and emails.

Practical Resources: From checklists to mental health exercises, we're bringing you practical resources that will turn the daunting into the doable.

Stories that Resonate: No more bland personality-less stories; you'll get stories from real people that resonate with you.

Upcoming Events and Webinars: Be the first to know about our webinars, live Q&A sessions, and events.

SCAN THE QR CODE TO ACCESS FREE BLOGS AND EMAILS

https://www.adultingwell.au/blogs

PART 2

PREPARING FOR SURGERY

CHAPTER

03

Mind Set

*"Surgery isn't happening to you,
it's happening for you!"*

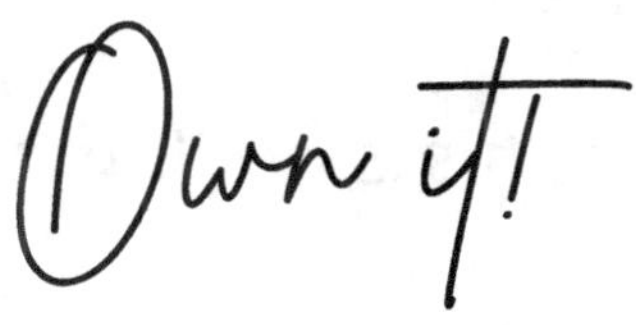

"You've really got to step into this and OWN IT! Yes, it's awful. No, it's not fair."

But it's going to happen, and you have the choice of how you want to get through to the other side. That choice all comes down to your mindset.

Your mindset is your guiding compass and your anchor through every moment of this journey.

Any idea that your surgery journey is out of your control couldn't be more wrong. It's not. You are not the passenger on this ride; you are in the driver's seat and in control. Take the wheel!

I'm not saying that you should think everything is sunshine and roses. I'm saying that it's okay to veer off course every now and then, but then you can take the wheel back because you're in control.

So, take charge of your mindset like never before. You hold the pen to write this chapter of your life, and it's going to be a chapter filled with practicality and success.

You are not defined by this surgery; you are defined by your mindset getting through it.

"Remember, this is not happening to you.

It's happening for you.

Own it!"

 **ACTION STEP:**
Write down what mindset
you are going to have for a
Successful Surgery

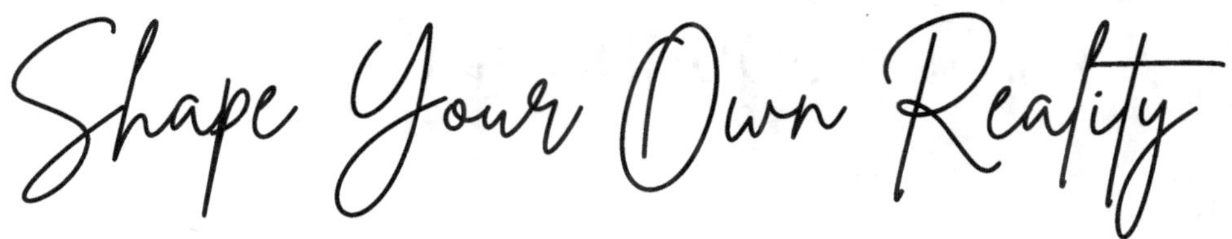

Shape Your Own Reality

You hold the power to shape your reality through your mindset. Once you've got a very clear idea of what that is, there are loads of ways to help you stay in the reality you want.

For this, you really only get out of it what you put in.

MEDITATION

Meditation and Hypnosis are some of the best ways to change and maintain your mindset. I used to think meditation was boring. But over the years, I've collected a bunch that really suit me and my style, and I'll bet there are ones that suit you, too.

 **TIP**: Here are some apps that I've used in the past:
- **Hypnosis Downloads** – An app by British psychologists. I recommend 'Easy with Needles', 'Prepare for Surgery' and ' Fast Natural Healing'. (https://www.hypnosisdownloads.com)
- **Headspace** – An Aussie app with practical exercises, breathing exercises, meditation, prompts to keep you on track and lots more. (https://www.headspace.com)
- **Calm** – A USA app with different types of meditation, breathing exercises, sleep stories, soundscapes, prompts and lots more. (https://www.calm.com)

JOURNALING

Carrying around all the thoughts and big emotions that come with preparing for major surgery is a heavy burden. Write that stuff down so it's out of your head, and you're not going around and around on the same points. You can word vomit all over the pages however you like. Your close friends and family will thank you because you'll be less inclined to word vomit all over them.

 **TIP**: Divide your page in half. On one half, write down how things are now for you. On the other side, write how you want things to be. Then, focus your energy on the positive side!

BREATHWORK

In the lead-up to surgery, I would get a whole bunch of nervous energy and wish I had ways to get rid of it. Exercise was definitely not an option pre-surgery, but I could have been doing breathwork. I fell into it a few years ago, and it's been a game-changer for me. I usually go into the session feeling a bit pent-up but come out every time feeling settled and more positive.

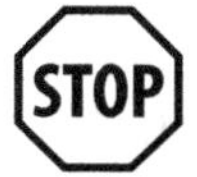 **Check with your medical professional before doing breathwork.**

OTHER

There are loads of other ways to shape your reality and stay in the mindset you want. You could do tapping, tai chi, or yoga. Art Therapy is also great. You can do things like painting, sculpting, colouring, music, and anything creative.

The goal is to find what works for you and be consistent with it.

ACTION STEP:
What strategies are you putting in place or continuing to shape your reality?

Mental Health Professional

I'll let you in on a secret. No one, and I mean no one, has all the strategies, tools, and coping mechanisms to face major surgery alone! I certainly didn't, and I've never met anyone who has.

This is where a professional comes in, someone who is trained in all the strategies, tools, and coping mechanisms you need.

A mental health professional, or as I like to call them - Mind Benders - have the tools you're gonna need in your toolkit to ace this.

Don't for a second think it's a sign of weakness to see a Mind Bender! You wouldn't become a professional athlete without a coach, would you? Hell no, you'd get the best damn coach you could! So why on earth would you think that you don't need a mental health professional to get you through major surgery? You do!

Your friends and family will be your biggest cheer squad. But chances are they are dealing with their own big feelings about seeing you go through this and may not be able to carry your big feelings as well.

Do them a favour and go see a Mind Bender. It is literally their job to listen to all your thoughts and feelings and work with you to build practical strategies, tools and coping mechanisms.

I'm not sure what else to say to convince you to see a Mind Bender. In my mind, there is no argument, no reason, no anything, not to do it. So go and get yourself a Mind Bender!

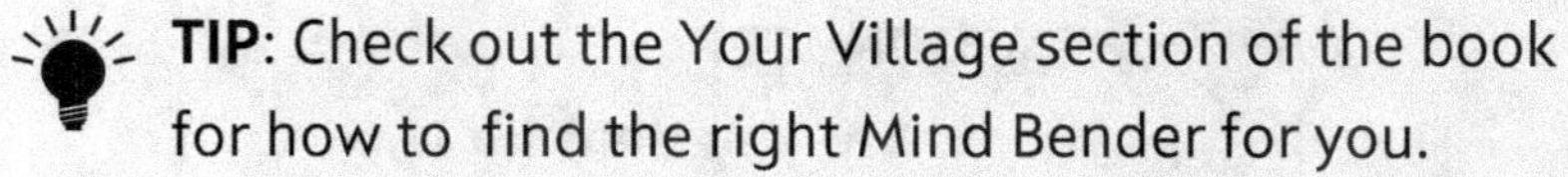

EXCESS BAGGAGE

For those of us who have been on the surgery journey a few times over now, you might have some excess baggage. I'm talking about trauma from previous hospital stints that might be catching up with you as you prep for this surgery.

Be super proactive about getting this in check. Talk to your Mind Bender, get coping mechanisms, and do the homework (strategies) to reduce, if not eliminate, this as you go in for this surgery. One surgery is enough without having to bring the baggage of your previous experiences as well.

"As I lined up for my 5th open heart surgery, I had a heck of a lot of baggage! I invested oodles of time with mind benders and doing the homework to resolve a lot of issues. Uncomfortable feelings and images still creep up on me sometimes, but its far less than it use to be and I have an awesome toolkit to dive into whenever I need. Don't suffer in silence. Get tools to sort it out now!"

<u>ACTION STEP:</u>
How are you dealing with your excess baggage?

Sleep

SLEEP ROUTINE

A good sleep routine is fundamental to keeping your mindset where you want. I get that it is so easy for me to write that sentence and an entirely different thing to do. But you can get a good night's sleep when you've got major surgery looming.

GET UP

Laying there alone at night gives your brain nothing but time to go over things. But there is a way to train it. Think of sleep like having a dog that you can train through positive reinforcement, distraction, and a few tricks. If you've been awake for more than 30 minutes, GET UP. Get yourself back to your anchor. If all else fails, distract yourself with something like TV.

MINDSET

Use the mindset that you wrote down as your anchor, keep circling back to it. Then double down on your homework – meditation, journaling, breathwork, and anything else. Also, lean into your Mind Bender to work through what's keeping you up.

 **TIP**: I've used a hypnosis called 'Night Worry' and the 'Insomnia Beater Pack' by Hypnosis Downloads for years and have found them very beneficial. (https://www.hypnosisdownloads.com)

 **ACTION STEP:**
What's your sleep routine?

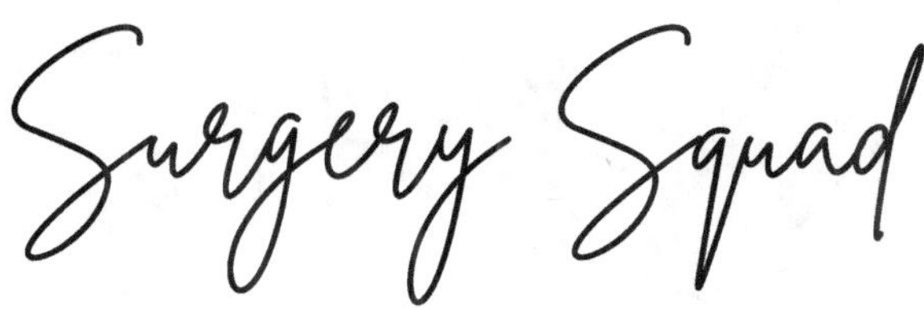

There is nothing more validating than talking to people who have experienced or are about to experience a similar surgery to you. I call this – finding your Surgery Squad.

SURGERY SQUAD

Community groups are fantastic! They provide a safe, moderated space to talk about your surgery and support others. I've asked questions about mindset, money, and how to talk to loved ones. I've also learnt so much from other people sharing.

Join the 'Adulting Well' Surgery Squad **by searching Facebook Community Groups.**

PODCASTS

Another booming way to stay connected with your Squad is through Podcasts.

The charity HeartKids has the podcast From the Heart, and yours truly has done a podcast called *'How to Prepare for Open-Heart Surgery... Tips and Tricks from a Pro!'* It's based on the first blog I wrote about going through surgery.

CHARITIES

There are over 600 charities dedicated to enhancing your surgery experience. They offer practical advice, understanding communities, and tailored support. Each charity has its unique approach, catering to your specific needs. Check the 'Your Village' section of this book for more details.

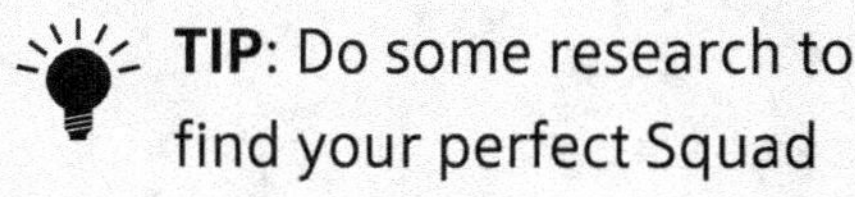

TIP: Do some research to find your perfect Squad

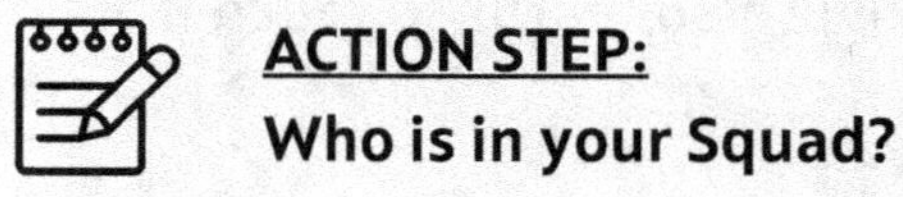

ACTION STEP:
Who is in your Squad?

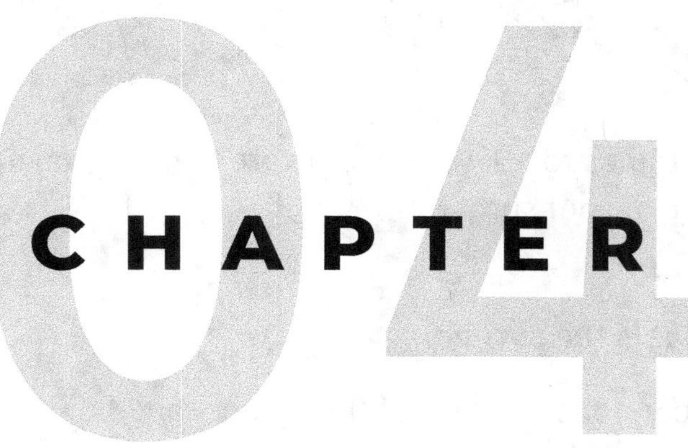

Pre-Game

*"Putting in the legwork
beforehand makes the world
of different post-surgery."*

Welcome to the pre-game, where we will gather some basic information that will be the building blocks for the rest of your surgery prep.

Surgery Questions

Here are 12 things to ask your healthcare team so you have a really clear picture of your surgery.

01 — What is the Surgery?

Understand the goal of the surgery and how it will address your health condition.

02 — When and where will the surgery be?

Confirm the exact date and hospital for the surgery. Sometimes, the exact date can't be set, so try just getting a ballpark date or month.

03 — What is the exact name of the device or implant?

Get the exact name of any devices or implants that are proposed, like the heart valve, hip joint, breast implant, or transplant - and details about how they work.

04 — What are the risks and benefits?

Discuss potential risks, complications, and side effects. Ask about potential long-term effects and outcomes.

05 — Are there alternatives?

Ask about any alternative treatments or procedures that might be available.

06 — What is the Anaesthesia Plan?

Understand the type of anaesthesia that will be used and how it might affect you during and after the surgery.

07   **Do I need to change medication before or after surgery?**

For some surgeries, you may need to change your current medication regime, and you may need different medication after the surgery.

08   **What are the Medicare Item Numbers?**

These codes identify and categorise medical services and procedures. They are crucial for understanding potential costs and insurance coverage.

09   **How much will it cost?**

Find out how much they expect the surgery and other services will cost.

10   **What Aftercare is Needed?**

Discuss post-surgery care instructions, including wound care, medication, and any lifestyle adjustments.

11   **What is the Recovery Time?**

Get an estimate of how long your recovery might take and what you can expect during that period.

12   **How long should I anticipate to be unable to work for?**

Get a guide on how long you will be unable to work or need to reduce your work effort.

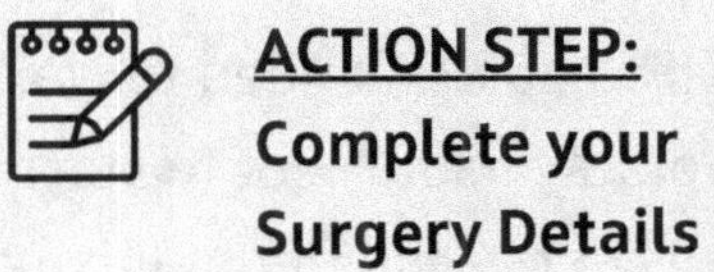

ACTION STEP:
**Complete your
Surgery Details**

PERSONAL QUESTIONS

It's time to equip yourself with the ultimate empowerment tool: a comprehensive list of questions that will leave no room for uncertainty.

No more sitting there dwelling on something you could get an answer to!

Get your Action Plan out, and whenever a question pops into your mind, whether it's at 2 a.m. or during your morning coffee, jot it down. Let your mind roam free and uncover every concern that's been on your radar. Think about the surgery and the recovery—there's no question too big or too small.

By giving yourself permission to explore these thoughts, you're paving the way for a clearer path ahead. As your list grows, so does your control over your own experience.

When you step into the surgeon's office, your list becomes your ally, ensuring no aspect is left unaddressed. So, let's get started – grab that pen, that device, or that notepad app, and let your questions flow freely.

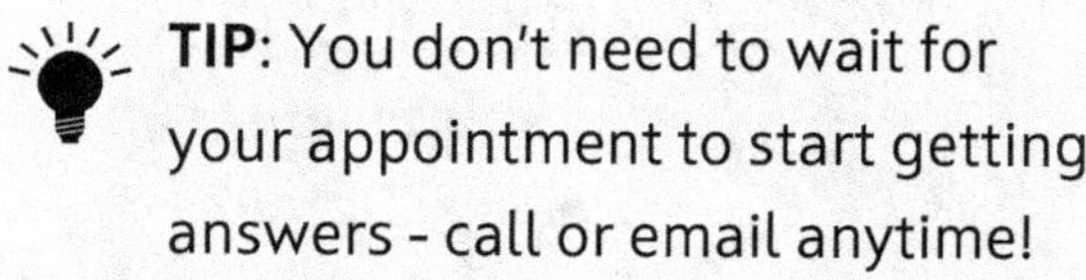

TIP: You don't need to wait for your appointment to start getting answers - call or email anytime!

"I had a very long list of questions and requests for my surgical team, like asking them not to secure my post-op breathing tube as tightly because last time, it pulled my lip. My surgeon was incredibly welcoming, even quipping, 'We don't usually get repeat customers.' The team did everything I requested and answered all my questions, which made the surgery much better."

ACTION STEP:
Write down all your questions and requests

Safety Briefing

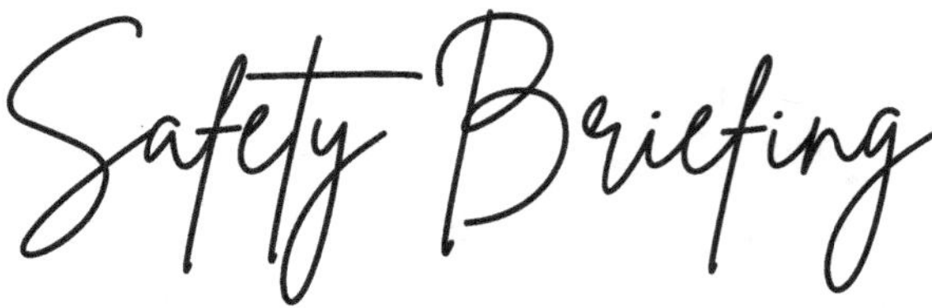

Up front, I want to say that major surgery now has the most rigorous safety measures in our history. Hospitals follow stringent protocols, and surgical teams conduct meticulous checklists to ensure no detail is overlooked.

Anaesthetists provide vigilant care during surgery, and infection control measures guard against potential threats. Our regulatory authority, the Therapeutic Goods Administration (TGA), rigorously evaluates medical devices, surgery tools, and medicines. The TGA safeguards your well-being, scrutinising quality, performance, safety, and efficacy. Hospitals and practitioners are also strictly governed.

Your safety is paramount, and Australia's meticulous processes stand as your steadfast guardians.

WHATS GOING INTO YOUR BODY

Once your medical team gives you the details about any devices or implants you are receiving, you can be a detective and find out more about them yourself.

The TGA in Australia is your go-to source for reliable and trusted information about specific medical devices and implants. You can search for your specific device using their online database, and you'll find detailed information about the device's approval status, specifications, and any safety alerts.

The TGA's commitment to safety and effectiveness is your ultimate guide in this digital age. So, gather knowledge and take charge of your health like never before.

To search your specific items, visit
https://www.tga.gov.au/resources/artg

 **TIP**: Your research might lead to more questions for your surgeon so jot them down in your action plan.

 **ACTION STEP:**
Research what devices you're getting and add them to your plan

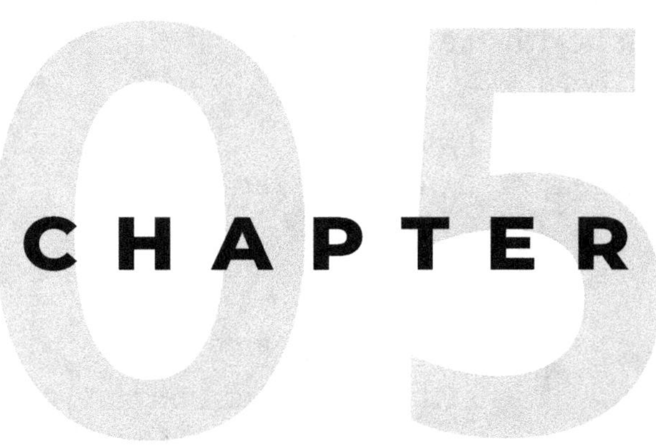

Your Village

"That saying, 'it takes a village' has never been more true than for getting through major surgery."

For Surgery Success, you'll need a village to support you, including a guardian angel, a GOAT, a Unicorn, a Surgery Squad, Bureaucrats, a Scrooge, and more.

Everyone in the village plays a part at some stage throughout your journey. You might not need them all at once, but you will need them at some stage. Find them early and have them in your back pocket whenever you need them.

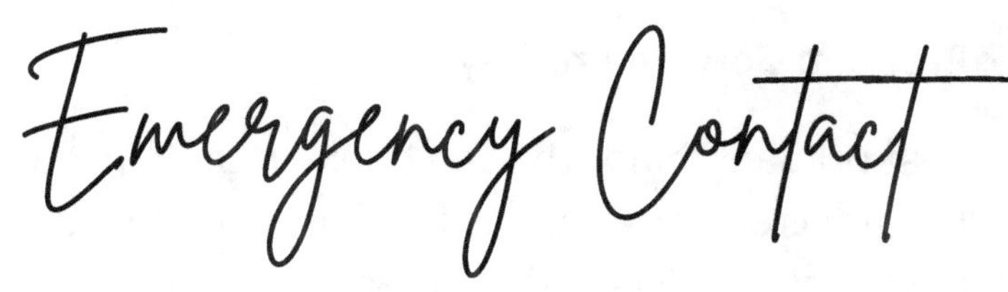

Guardian Angel

Who is your "Guardian Angel," your emergency contact and next of kin? Who will come to your aid when you need it the most?

Take a moment to identify this special person and have a heartfelt conversation with them about what you might need in case of an emergency. You'll need this person (and their deets) for everything! From hospital paperwork, a shoulder to lean on, right through to letting your workplace know.

Level up your preparedness by choosing a second Guardian Angel who's ready to step in, too. Trust me, having a dynamic duo will save the day.

THE BEST GUARDIAN ANGELS

01 **Swift Responder Extraordinaire**

Someone who can leap into action at a moment's notice! A quick phone call away, they'll race to your side when you need them most.

02 **Calm and Collected Comforter**

Someone with a soothing presence who can keep the chaos at bay. With their calming words and reassuring smiles, they'll be your ultimate source of comfort.

Problem-Solving Prodigy

03

That brilliant mind who can think on their feet and come up with creative solutions in a flash! They'll navigate any unexpected twists and turns with ease.

Anchor

04

Someone with unwavering reliability and steadfastness! They'll be the anchor in your life, always there to lend a helping hand and offer unwavering support.

Positive Energy Powerhouse

05

That ray of sunshine who brings positivity wherever they go! With their infectious optimism, they'll brighten your darkest days and turn challenges into opportunities for growth.

Mental Health Professional

Mind Bender

A mental health professional—or, as I like to call them, Mind Benders—has the tools you'll need in your toolkit to ace this. Check out the 'Mindset' chapter for why.

THE RIGHT MIND BENDER FOR YOU

Finding the right Mind Bender is a bit like dating. You really need to hit it off and have a great rapport. If you don't, you can politely decline a second date (i.e. session), then contact the provider and get a different person or find someone else yourself.

 **TIP:** You'll probably already be out of your comfort zone staring down the face of surgery, so find someone who helps you get comfortable and gives you practical ways to deal with everything.

There are so many ways to find a Mind Bender these days. There really is no excuse not to have one. Below are some of the most common ways to find one, but there might be other ways as well.

EMERGENCY SUPPORT

If you ever need emergency support, call one of these organisations. They are ready to take your call—most of them 24 hours a day—and they are all free.

Emergency mental health contacts:
LifeLine 13 11 14
Sane 1800 18 7263
Beyond Blue 1300 22 4636
MensLine 1300 789 978
Suicide Call Back Service 1300 659 467

 **TIP**: Sometimes Mind Benders take a bit of time to get into, so these are a fantastic alternatives.

MENTAL HEALTH CARE PLAN

If your General Practitioner (GP) or specialist diagnose you with a mental health condition, they can create a special Mental Health Care Treatment Plan with you for treatment options and support services. This plan includes a set number of sessions with a Mental Health Professional.

The plan is not a blank cheque to see any Mind Bender. Each

Mind Bender sets their own fees, so Medicare may only cover some of the cost. Ask how much you'll pay and what you'll get back from Medicare when you make your appointment.

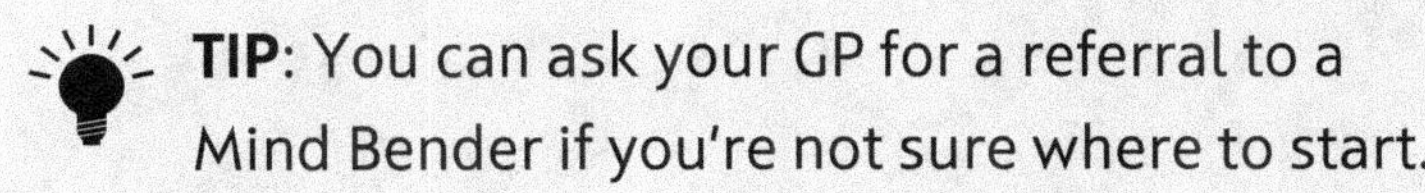

EMPLOYEE ASSISTANCE PROGRAM (EAP)

I love EAP! It's free access to a Mind Bender through your workplace. Each workplace arranges EAP in its own way. The suite of services provided by any EAP will include free Mind Bender sessions for you and your family (separately or together). Some EAPs also offer career coaching, support for managers, financial counselling, and more.

To find out if you have access, check your work's intranet, call Human Resources, or ask around. It's free and confidential. Whatever you say to them, they won't pass it on to your employer; it's just between you and them.

ON YOUR OWN

You can also go it alone and find your own Mind Bender. To find one, you can check this national database of counsellors:

https://www.healthdirect.gov.au/australian-health-services

Doing it this way means that you'll need to do your own research, weigh up your needs, determine the payment pathway and sort it out.

*"Don't let this deter you! I've found
a couple of counsellors this way,
and they have helped me change
my life. Most great ones I've found
through word of mouth."*

BOOKING

Sometimes, getting in to see your Mind Bender can take longer than you'd like. It happens to all of us. Hang in there it will be worth the wait.

 **TIP**: Pre-book multiple Mind Bender sessions before your surgery, and a couple for afterwards.

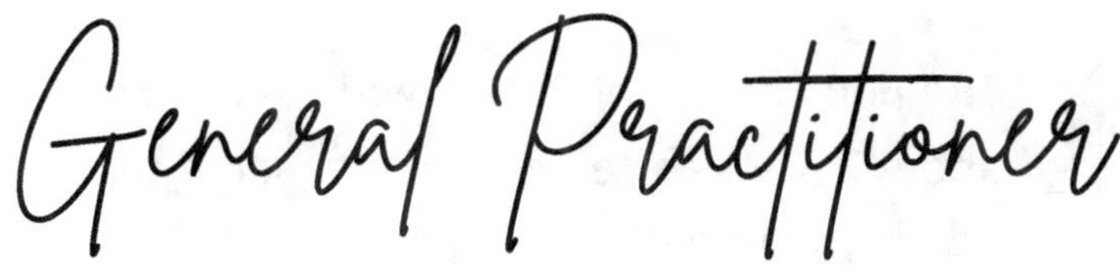

Unicorn

The right GP is like a Unicorn. They are rare and absolutely magnificent in person but damn hard to find. There are plenty of horses (regular GPs), but that unicorn (special GP) who has an interest or training in your condition is pure gold. When you find them, hold onto them with both hands.

Unicorns are the frontline for almost everything medical you'll need. They do referrals to specialists, help with mental health access and medications, and help you manage your condition day-to-day.

UNICORN HUNTING

Top 3 ways to find a Unicorn:

01   **Family and Friends**

Recommendations from those nearest and dearest.

02   **Online Directories**

HealthDirect service finder:
https://www.healthdirect.gov.au/australian-health-services

03   **Local Health Clinics and Hospitals**

Google search clinics and hospitals in your area.

 **TIP**: Book an appointment with your GP for about 2 weeks after your home just in case you need anything. You can always cancel it.

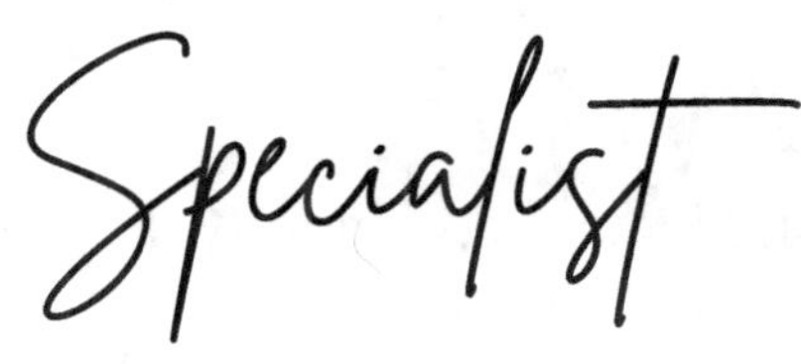

G.O.A.T

Specialists are the shizzle, the OG, and the GOAT! That's the Original Gangster (OG) and Greatest of All Time (GOAT). So don't mess about it; go and get yourself a GOAT.

Your GOAT isn't just a medical expert; they're like your health BFF. They know your struggles, your quirks, and your health dreams. They craft a plan that's as unique as you are, making sure you get the VIP treatment you deserve.

Their knowledge is like a security blanket for your health. No more Googling your symptoms at 2 a.m. and ending up convinced you have a rare tropical disease! With your GOAT, you can rest easy knowing you've got a top-notch expert watching over you.

GOAT HUNTING

Top 3 ways to find a GOAT:

01   **Referrals**

Your GP can refer you to a specialist.

02   **Online Directories**

HealthDirect service finder:
https://www.healthdirect.gov.au/australian-health-services

03

Word of Mouth

Ask around in your community groups.

64

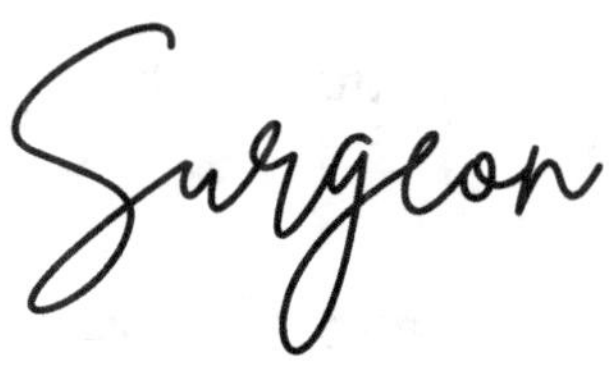

The Artist

Your surgeon plays a crucial role in your major surgery. They use their tools with precision to make life-changing improvements to your health.

They can reshape, repair, and restore your body. They understand it deeply, having studied its unique characteristics and planned the transformation carefully.

You should feel free to share your concerns with your surgeon. They are there to collaborate with you, combining their expertise with your hopes for the future.

ARTIST HUNTING

Top 4 ways to find an Artist:

01 **Referrals**

From your Unicorn (GP) or GOAT (Specialist).

02 **Online Directories**

HealthDirect service finder:
https://www.healthdirect.gov.au/australian-health-services

03 **Hospital Referrals**

If you're going through the public healthcare system, you

might not have the option to choose your surgeon.

Private Health Insurance Network

If you have private health insurance, you'll likely have the choice of which Artist you want. Check your insurer's network and find specialists who are covered by your plan.

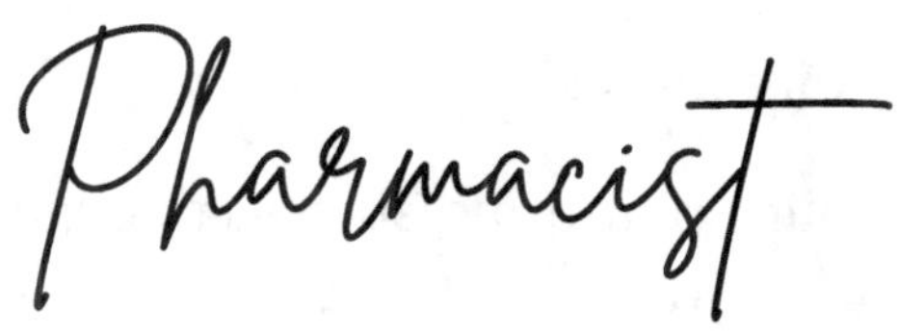

The Alchemist

Your Alchemist is your go-to for deciphering medication instructions, managing potential interactions, and addressing any concerns about side effects. With their guidance, you'll navigate the path of prescriptions with confidence.

Your Alchemist isn't just a dispenser of pills; they're your partners in understanding and managing your medications effectively. They can also help you out with the odd medical certificate. Don't hesitate to reach out to them for guidance and support.

ALCHEMIST HUNTING

Top 3 Ways to Find Your Alchemist:

01

Local Pharmacies

Your local community pharmacy is often full of expertise.

02

Hospital Pharmacies

They work closely with your medical team to ensure proper medication management and administration during your stay.

Online Directories

Many online platforms, such as the Pharmacy Guild of Australia's directory, offer a convenient way to find reputable Alchemists in your area. You can search by location or specialty to find a pharmacist who suits your needs.

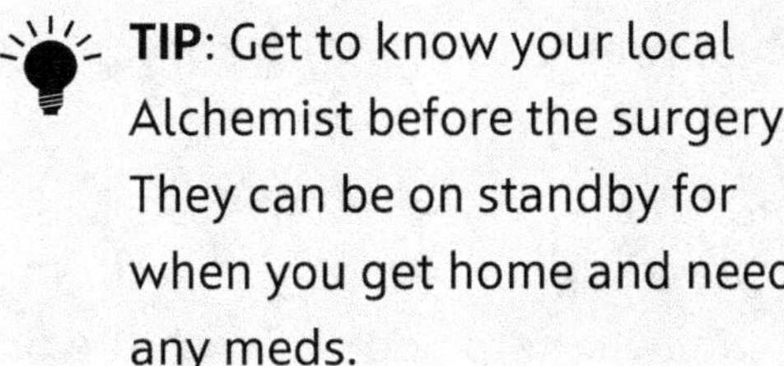

TIP: Get to know your local Alchemist before the surgery. They can be on standby for when you get home and need any meds.

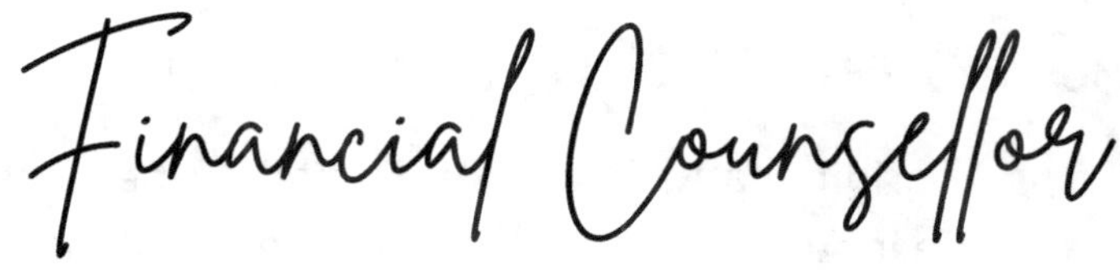

Financial Counsellor

Scrooge

There are free Scrooges! And they're here to team up with you for your major surgery. First off, Scrooge can help you whip up a budget that's surgery-ready. They'll walk you through every cost, making sure you're prepared for whatever comes your way. Scrooge is your guide to uncovering hidden government and other benefits, making sure you're not missing out on any financial support.

Insurance talk can be confusing, but fear not! Scrooge speaks the language of insurance companies and helps you decode the jargon. They make sure you're getting the most out of your coverage, leaving no stone unturned. Scrooge can step in to help you navigate the debt maze. They're experts at negotiating, consolidating, and lightening the financial load so you can focus on your surgery journey.

SCROOGE HUNTING

Top 3 Ways to Find Your Scrooge:

01 **National Debt Helpline at 1800 007 007**

Helps anyone tackle their debt problems.

02 **Mob Strong Debt Helpline at 1800 808 488**

Helps Aboriginal and Torres Strait Islander peoples from anywhere in Australia with legal advice and financial counselling.

03 **Small Business Debt Helpline at 1800 413 828**

Helps small business owners struggling with finances.

04 **Rural Financial Counselling Service Program at 1300 771 741**

Helps farmers, fishing enterprises, forestry growers and harvesters, and small related businesses experiencing, or at risk of, financial hardship.

05 **Employee Assistance Programs (EAP)**

Some workplaces offer Employee Assistance Programs (EAP), including financial counselling services. Check yours out; it might surprise you.

These are all free services. You can also find paid services on your own.

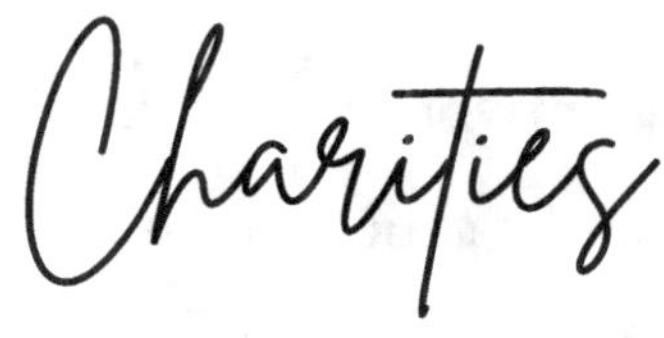

Champions

There are over 600 charities working in the health sector ready to be your champion!

These organisations are dedicated to bringing a unique perspective to your surgery path. They're not just sources of information; they're your partners in empowerment, offering practical advice, understanding ears, and a community that resonates with your experience.

CHAMPION HUNTING

A few awesome charities waiting to be your champion:

01 **Heart Foundation**

Offers valuable resources and support for adults facing major surgery related to heart conditions.

02 **HeartKids**

The only charity dedicated to people with childhood-onset heart disease (like me). They have a helpline and resources, including my surgery blog.

03 **Cancer Council Australia**

For adults undergoing major surgery due to cancer.

04   **Breast Cancer Network Australia**

Your ally for breast cancer surgery in Australia.

05   **Rare Cancers Australia**

For adults undergoing major surgery for a rare cancer.

06   **Lung Foundation Australia**

A guiding light for adults navigating major lung-related surgeries.

07   **Endometriosis Australia**

For women undergoing major surgery due to endometriosis.

08   **Australian Red Cross**

Offers a helping hand to adults facing any major surgery.

09   **Angel Flight Australia**

It provides a vital lifeline for adults needing to travel long distances for major surgery.

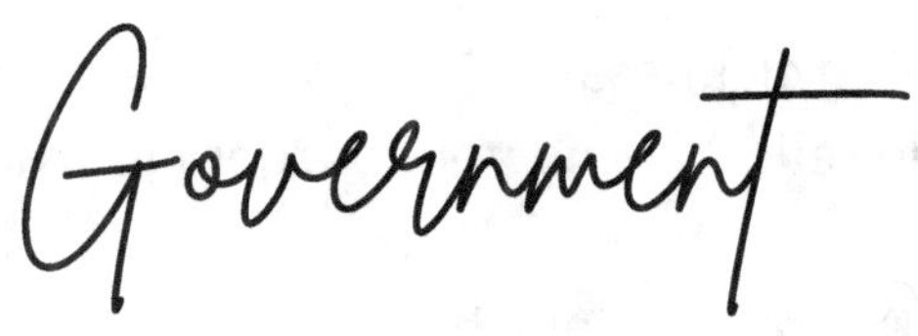

Bureaucrats

Each bureaucrat (i.e. Government agency) brings its own expertise and approach tailored to address your specific needs and concerns. Whether you're seeking financial aid, medical information, or logistical support, there's an agency to assist you.

Government responsibilities are divided between state and federal levels. The Feds (Federal government) handle national matters like Medicare and broader health policies. While state governments manage matters like healthcare services within state-owned hospitals. All the bureaucrats collaborate to ensure a holistic approach to your care and support.

BURAEUCRAT HUNTING

Four government agencies you should know about:

01 **Medicare**
Medicare is your health safety net. With their comprehensive coverage, they ensure that you have access to necessary medical services and support.

02 **Centrelink**
Centrelink offers a range of financial support services,

03

Departments of Health

These agencies (state and federal) provide crucial information and resources related to health services, medical research, and healthcare policies.

04

National Disability Insurance Scheme (NDIS)

NDIS is here to support people with disabilities, including some of us facing major surgery.

Employer
the Boss

Your Boss can be your advocate, understanding your needs and providing the necessary support to ensure your work-life balance remains intact. Chatting with "The Boss" makes for a win-win situation. Sharing your surgery plans, recovery timeline, and any adjustments you might require lays the groundwork for a smooth journey ahead.

It's not just about transition; it's about building trust and synergy between work and well-being.

 **TIP**: Check out the 'Work' chapter for more details on how to work with your Boss.

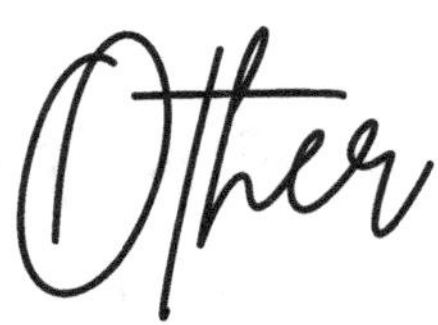

There are so many others that you can have as part of your village.

01 Physiologist or Exercise Physiologist

They create personalised exercise plans to safely improve strength, flexibility, and overall fitness, aiding surgery preparation, recovery and symptom management.

02 Nutritionist or Dietician

Offers tailored dietary plans to support your body before and after surgery, enhancing recovery and boosting your overall health.

03 Massage Therapist

A massage therapist can support you before and after surgery by easing muscle tension, improving circulation, and promoting relaxation, which aids in both preparation and recovery. Some private health insurance cover this.

04 Allied Health Professionals

This includes professionals like; occupational therapists, speech therapists, podiatrists, and social workers. They offer specialised support to address various needs before and after surgery, enhancing your overall care and recovery.

05 Hospitals

Hospitals and their key staff, including anaesthetists,

nurses, and medical coordinators, ensure you receive comprehensive care, expert treatment, and effective management throughout your surgery and recovery process.

Home Care Provider

These very special people offer practical assistance with daily living activities, such as personal care, household chores, and meal preparation, helping to ease the burden and support your preparation and recovery at home.

Lawyer or Legal Aid

A lawyer can assist with estate planning, wills, power of attorney, and advanced care directives. They can also help navigate disability rights, insurance claims, and medical malpractice issues, ensuring your rights and interests are protected.

Family and Friends

Family and friends offer emotional support, practical help, and companionship, making your preparation and recovery smoother and less isolating.

Children's School

School staff, including teachers, year coordinators, and support personnel, can provide crucial assistance with your child's education and well-being during your surgery and recovery, offering accommodations and understanding.

Add anyone else you think you may need into your Village.

Facing major surgery can be overwhelming, but having a strong support village makes a big difference. Relying on these people helps you manage the practical aspects of your surgery, from daily tasks to emotional support, ensuring you navigate the process more smoothly and effectively.

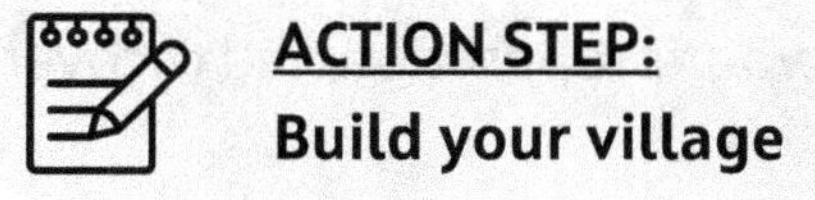
ACTION STEP:
Build your village

CHAPTER

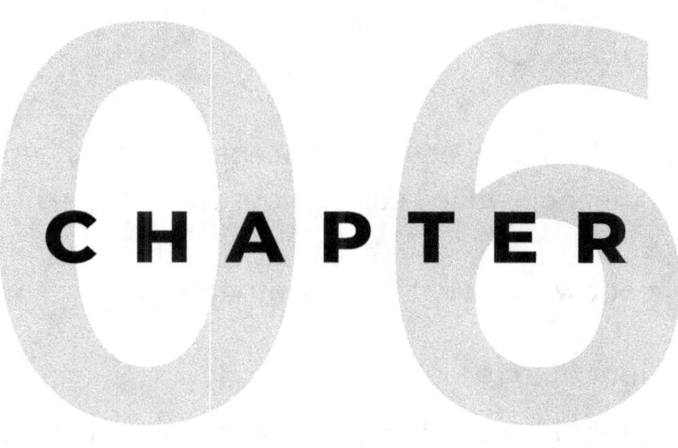

Crowd Control

"The people in my life helped make all of my surgeries as good as they were."

As you prepare for surgery, there are loads of people who want to support you. So much so that it can get overwhelming. This is where you need some practical ways to control the crowd of well-wishers. From crafting the perfect Coms Plan to keep everyone in the loop to deciding who gets a backstage pass to the hospital and beyond, you're about to become a pro at crowd control.

Coms Plan

A top-notch Coms Plan keeps your peeps – friends, fam, and work buddies – in the loop while keeping your vibe and privacy intact.

Here's the lowdown on what to toss into the mix:

01 The Inner Circle

Time to round up your go-to people, your inner circle. Think immediate family, BFFs, and even some work buddies. They get the VIP updates straight from you.

02 Virtual Updates

For your broader social network, embrace technology by setting up an exclusive email list or private group on your fave social media platform.

03 Spokesperson

Be a pro and get a spokesperson who's got your back when it comes to answering everyone's questions or concerns. They'll give updates on your behalf, repeat the same info to different people, and generally keep the crowd in control.

04 Regular Updates

How often do you want to give updates? Some people prefer daily or weekly messages, while others might opt for key milestones or important developments. Your spokesperson can do them for you until you can do them yourself.

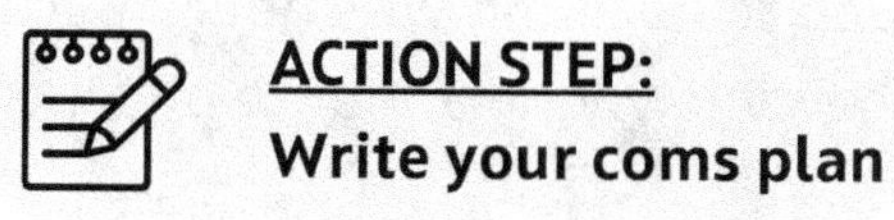

ACTION STEP:
Write your coms plan

Visitors

The decision to have visitors in the hospital and during recovery might not steal headlines, but it actually makes a pretty big impact. Making this decision early means you'll have clear boundaries, and it won't be yet another decision you need to make in between meds, travel, and everything else.

Here are a couple of things to factor in when making this decision:

01 Health

Prioritise your health and recovery, and consider whether visitors might compromise your well-being or expose you to infections.

02 Medical Recommendations

Consult your healthcare team for advice on whether having visitors aligns with your recovery plan and medical condition.

03 Comfort Zone

Reflect on your personal comfort level with having visitors, weighing the benefits of their presence against your need for rest and solitude.

04 Visitor Policy

Understand the hospital's visitor policies, especially in relation to infection control measures or restrictions due to health crises.

"I've gone both ways with either having loads of visitors or just the inner circle. Having just the inner circle and spokesperson to keep everyone else updated worked the best for me. I could just focus on healing and celebrating the small wins. When I felt stronger, I caught up with everyone."

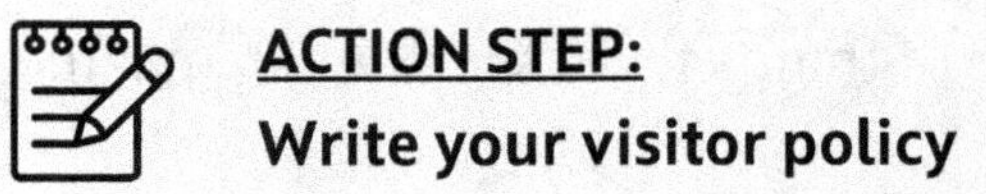

ACTION STEP:
Write your visitor policy

Emergency Contact

Check out the 'Your Village' section of the book for details about your Emergency Contact and the qualities to look for in picking the right person.

So you are both on the same page, check out the script below you could use to kick-off a chat with them about your surgery.

Hey, I wanted to talk to you about something important. As you know, I have surgery coming up, and I'm very grateful for your support. I know this might be new for both of us, so I think it will be handy for us to be on the same page. I want you to know that I value your help deeply.

I also get that this might be a bit overwhelming for you as well. So let's approach this as a team. We're in this together, and I truly believe that by setting some goals, we can make things smoother.

I was thinking that having a schedule or routine could be beneficial. I know surgery can be unpredictable, but having a general plan for meals, medications, and rest could give us some structure.

Another thing I'd like to suggest is having a designated time each day or week to check-in. We can talk about how we're feeling and any concerns we might have, and even celebrate the small victories. It'll help us stay connected and up to speed.

(continues on next page)

Communication is key for me, so I'd like us to promise to talk openly about how things are going. If something feels overwhelming or if we need to adjust our approach, I want us to feel comfortable discussing it without any judgment.

Lastly, I want to acknowledge that this experience could be stressful for both of us. Let's remember that it's okay to feel a range of emotions. Seeing a mental health professional, together or separately, would be good for each of us.

Thank you for being here with me. Your support means the world to me, and I know that with a plan in place and a positive attitude, we can face this surgery together.

ACTION STEP:
Make notes and have the chat with your Emergency Contact

Note Takers

I just wanted to make a special note about having a note-taker with you at appointments.

It's no secret that appointments can sometimes feel overwhelming, and absorbing all the information might be challenging. That's where a note-taker comes in to help you out. With someone jotting down the details, you can engage fully in the discussion without worrying about forgetting a crucial point.

After the appointment, you and your note-taker can revisit the conversation and clarify any uncertainties. This lets you digest the information at your own pace, ensuring that no critical details are missed or misconstrued. It's a practical way to empower yourself and enhance your understanding of your healthcare journey.

"We've established a helpful tradition for my appointments – having a dedicated note-taker. It used to be my mum, and now my husband has taken up the role. He walks in with his phone ready, notes app open, and starts typing away! After the appointment, we head to a nearby café to review and discuss the notes. This practice has been a game-changer, allowing me to concentrate on asking my questions instead of stressing about remembering every detail shared during the appointment."

Communicating with Kids

If you're a parent, this bit is just for you! Juggling the roles of patient and parent requires some planning, open communication, and a splash of creativity.

9 TIPS TO MANAGE THE KIDS

Your little ones are undoubtedly your top priority, so here are some things to think about and plan for as you navigate surgery and recovery.

01

Childcare Arrangements

First things first—lining up who's on duty while you're off duty. Whether it's the grandparents, trusted friends, or lovely neighbours, find your squad who can tag in while you're in the hospital and recovering.

02

Open Communication

Simplify the surgery explanation for your kids. Use language they understand to explain that you'll have a procedure to feel better. Assure them that doctors and nurses will care for you, and you'll be back home soon. If you need help with this, there are some scripts below.

03

Behaving Differently

As a result of the surgery or any other treatment, you might end up behaving differently than your kids are used to - tell them that this might happen. You could be more

03
tired, not feel up to playing, not be up for doing the school run, and want more chill time on the couch with them than normal. Let them know all of this.

04
Keep the Routine Rollin'

Mini humans thrive on routine, so give your caregiver the lowdown on your kid's daily routine. Share the details – meal times, play dates, and lights-out times. A well-maintained routine means a little less chaos.

05
Create a Comforting Environment

Sending your kiddo off with a familiar comfort item–like a snuggly blanket or a plushie–can make all the difference. It's like a little piece of you tagging along, giving them a warm hug when you can't be there.

06
Coms Plan

Staying in touch is a must. Set up a game plan with your caregiver on how to keep the lines open. Whether it's video chats that'll make you both laugh or quick texts to swap stories, a little connection goes a long way.

07
The Reunion Talk

After the surgery, your kids might wonder where you've been. Keep it simple and honest–let them know you need a bit of help to get better. Explain that you're home sweet home now and what they can expect from you.

08
Quality Time

As you start to feel better, embrace the precious moments with your kids. Dive into cozy reading sessions, have movie marathons, or have a board game showdowns.

09

The Power of "Yes, Please!":

Don't hesitate to let others lend a hand. If friends offer to whip up dinner or help with laundry, say "yes!" Accepting help not only eases your load but lets your kids see the wonderful village of support surrounding your family.

Not sure how to explain your surgery to your kids? Try some of these words:

For 2-5 year olds:

Mum/Dad is going to the hospital for a little while, but it's all to make sure I feel better. You know how we visit the doctor when you have a boo-boo? Well, I'm going to see special doctors who have the tools to help fix something inside my body.

Just like when we visit the doctor, they'll take care of me and make sure everything is working just right. I'll miss you while I'm away, but it won't be gone for long. When I come back home, I might need some extra rest to get better. I might be a bit different. But, we can plan things to do for when I'm better.

For 5-10 year olds:

I'm going to the hospital for a little while. You know how our bodies have different parts that work together; well, one part of my body needs a little fixing, and the fantastic doctors at the hospital will help make it better. They will use their special tools and skills to make everything work perfectly.

I might stay in the hospital for a bit, but I'll be with people who care about me and want to help me feel great again. After resting for about xx days/weeks, I'll be back home. Then I'll need a bit more rest and might act a bit differently before I'm ready for our next big adventure together!

For 10-15 year olds:

You know how sometimes things in life need a bit of fixing or tweaking to work better? Well, that's what's happening with me. I'm going to the hospital for a surgery. It's like a team of experts getting together to make sure my body is in top-notch shape. Just like how we troubleshoot and upgrade our gadgets, the doctors are going to do the same for me.

It's totally okay to have questions or feel curious about it—ask me anything. I'm going to be in the hospital for xx days/weeks, but I'll have people taking care of me and checking in on me every step of the way. Then I'll be back home and still need a bit of time to recover, so I might act a bit differently before diving back into all our fun stuff.

For 15-20 year olds:

I'm going to have a surgery, which might sound a bit intense, but it's all about making sure my body stays strong and healthy. Think of it like a maintenance check for a car – sometimes you need to give it a tune-up to keep it running smoothly. The doctors and medical team are experts at what they do, and they're going to work their magic to make sure everything's shipshape.

I'll be in the hospital for xx days/weeks, but I've got a support squad around me, and they're going to make sure I'm comfortable and well taken care of. When I get home I'll need a bit more time to recover and might act a bit differently. If you've got any questions or thoughts, feel free to ask – I appreciate your understanding and support.

ACTION STEP:
Make a plan for your kids
and have a chat with them

Communicating with Mates

Have a chat with your mates about what you're going through. They probably need help understanding the in's and out's of your health, and the only way they will is if you TELL THEM!

I get it—you don't want to be a burden on your mates. But trust me, you're not. True friends are there for the good and the bad times. Telling them gives you a chance to figure out how you want to be supported and them a chance to figure out how they can best support you. It goes both ways.

Let them know if you're trying to manage physical symptoms before surgery. This will help them understand if you have to reduce the time you spend with them or change how you hang out.

Surgery can also be a big mental load, so it's good to let them know how you're coping with it mentally. In dealing with all the things that major surgery throws at you, chances are your behaviour might change. Letting your mates know what you're feeling can help them find the best ways to support you and not be surprised or confused if/when you act out of character.

If you don't tell people what's happening and they notice changes in your behaviour, they will naturally fill the knowledge gap with their own story.

 **TIP:** Your mates are likely not fully trained therapists, so try striking a balance between leaning on them for support and getting professional help when you need it.

"Pre-surgery, I was always fatigued and could only do low-energy activities with friends, like watching a movie. I didn't always explain this well, which led to some friends being confused and thinking I didn't want to spend time with them. Learning to explain my mental and physical state has made all my friendships stronger."

Not sure how to bring up the subject of your surgery with your mate, try this:

I'm having major surgery soon, and I thought it would be good to let you know what's going on. I'm feeling a bit nervous about it, and I could really use your support during this time.

Physically, I might be dealing with a lot of fatigue and discomfort, so I may not have as much energy or time to hang out as usual. Please know that if I need to cancel plans or only do low-energy activities, it's not because I don't want to spend time with you.

Mentally, this surgery is a big load to carry, and there might be times when I seem different or act out of character. I've got some great resources and am doing everything I can to cope well.

I don't want to overwhelm you or turn our conversations into therapy sessions, but sharing this with you helps me feel more at ease. Your support and just knowing you're there for me would be a huge comfort. Thanks!

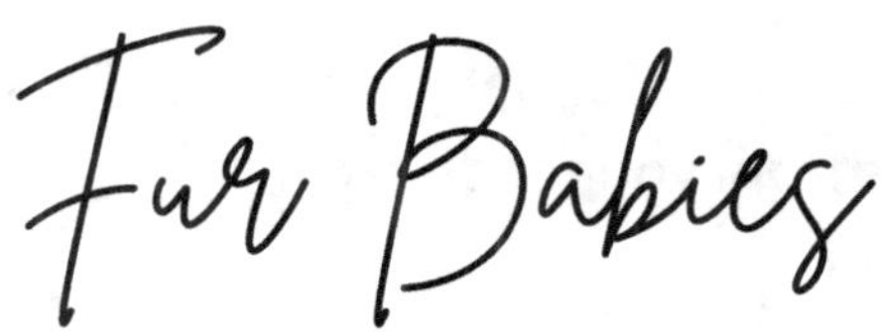

Fur Babies

Let's not forget our furry, fluffy, scaly or feathered family members! They might not understand all the medical stuff, but they sure know when something's up. Here are some tips to keep your fur babies happy while you're on the mend:

01

Pet-sitter

Find a trusted friend, family member, or pet-sitting service to take care of your fur baby while you're away. Make sure they're well-fed, walked, and cuddled.

02

Virtual Cuddles

Set up video calls with your fur baby. They might not quite get the whole screen thing, but they'll definitely recognise your voice and feel your love.

Comfort Zone

03

Leave behind some of your clothing or a blanket that smells like you. Your scent can be a source of comfort for them while you're not around.

04

Treat Central

Prep some special treats or toys in advance for your fur baby to enjoy. It's like a surprise party they'll love!

Updates and Pics

05

Have your pet-sitter send you photos and updates so you

05 can see how your fur baby is doing. It's like getting postcards from your pet's vacation.

And when you're back home, remember to manage the fur-tastic reunion! After surgery, you might not be up for your fur baby's enthusiastic jump-a-thon. It's a good idea to have a plan in place for the grand return.

Maybe designate a cuddle zone where they can chill without the acrobatics and gradually reintroduce them to your lap as you feel better. That way, you'll both have a smoother transition back to your regular snuggle sessions.

"I didn't really think this through, and my gorgeous cat definitely knew something was up when I got home from surgery and tried to comfort me by sitting as close to my chest as he could. Not ideal. He was less than impressed when my husband collected him, but it was short-lived, and I was up for furry cuddles soon enough."

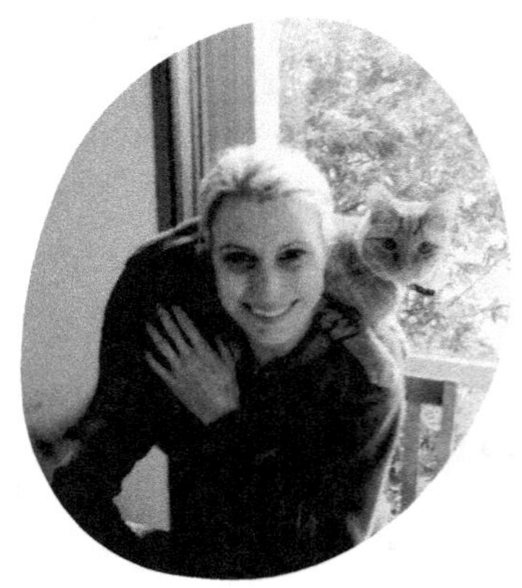

2011 - 28 Years Old - Oscar and I living our best lives

ACTION STEP:
Make your Fur Baby Plan

CHAPTER

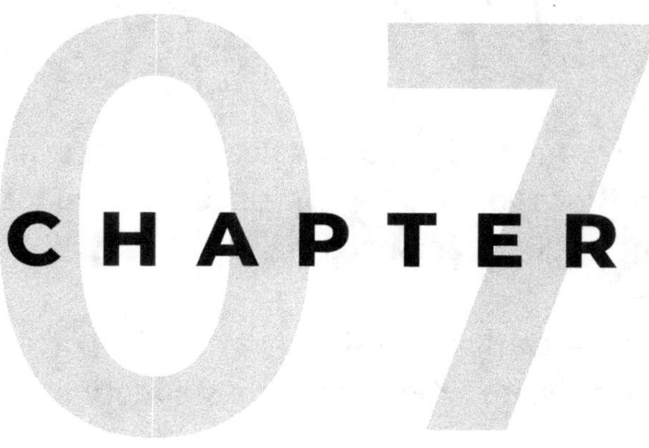

"Healthcare can be costly, but after four decades of managing these expenses, I've discovered the most effective and budget-friendly hacks you need to know."

This part is a bit dense. I get that money can be overwhelming when you're unwell! Or really, anytime. But before you put this book down or skip this part, just know that it's all beautifully chunked down for you. By the end of this part you'll know all the financial ins and outs, what your options are, and have a plan to get through it all. Yes, we're gonna budget! Yay (I love this stuff).

Medical Expenses

Have you ever wondered about the finances of the medical world down under? Brace yourself for some eye-opening facts and figures to put it all into perspective.

In Australia, our healthcare system is a massive force of nature. Our annual healthcare expenditure is a staggering $185 billion!

With more than 2.5 million surgeries annually, our hospitals are bustling hubs of activity. Aussies also make around 178 million visits to various medical practitioners. It's like having the entire population of Australia (25 million people), plus a few million friends, visiting the doctor's office every year.

And let's not forget our Medicare system, which shelled out $24 billion in benefits just last year, ensuring our fellow Aussies get the care they need without breaking the bank.

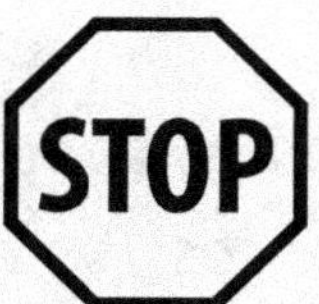

The information in this Book is not Financial Advice.

You are encouraged to seek formal advice and to read the disclaimer and terms and conditions of this Book.

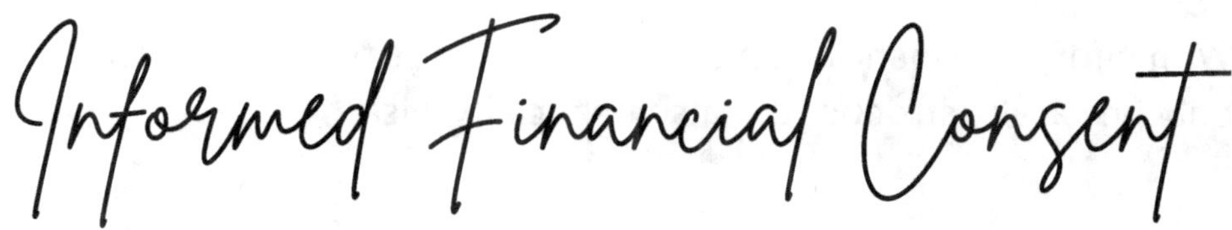

Informed Financial Consent

Informed Financial Consent is here to make sure you're not hit with any surprise bills post-surgery.

Australian law requires healthcare providers to be crystal clear about the costs involved in your treatment. Yes, it's literally the law that you know how much this will cost you.

Here's a list of things you could be charged for:

- Surgeon fees
- Anaesthetist fees
- Specialist fees
- Hospital accommodation
- Operating theatre costs
- Medication costs
- Diagnostic tests (e.g., X-rays, MRI)
- Pathology fees
- Prosthetics or implants
- Post-operative care costs
- Rehabilitation costs

Not sure how to have the money conversation with your Village? Try this:

I wanted to discuss the potential costs associated with my upcoming surgery.

Could you provide me with a breakdown of all the expenses, including any out-of-pocket costs?

Understanding the financial aspect will help me better prepare for the procedure and make informed decisions about my healthcare.

With Informed Financial Consent, you'll emerge from surgery not only physically stronger but also financially wiser.

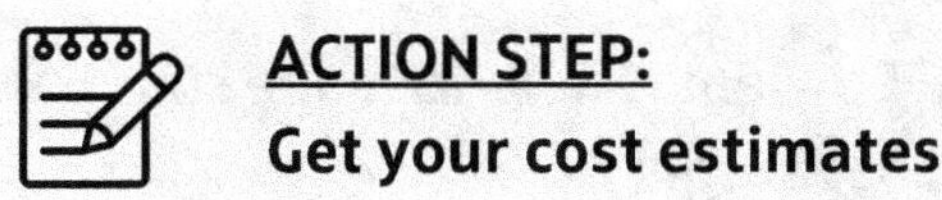

Ballpark Medical Costs

Say hello to your new BFF - the Medical Cost Finder! This nifty online tool is like your surgery budgeting guru, helping you figure out your potential medical expenses.

Just visit the **Medical Costs Finder,** punch in the type of surgery you're having or those magical Medicare Item Numbers, and voilà!

You'll get a ballpark figure of what you might expect to pay.

Medical Cost Finder:
https://medicalcostsfinder.health.gov.au/search

 **TIP**: To make the most of this tool, keep details handy, such as the type of procedure, relevant Medicare Item Number/s, and private health insurance details.

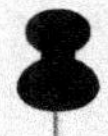 **NOTE:** The tool only offers *estimates* based on general data. So, think of it as an insight, not the ultimate oracle for your medical expenses.

 **ACTION STEP:**
Get your ballpark medical costs (crosscheck with what you found out earlier from your Village)

Medicare

Australia's Medicare system is a federal government-run marvel that provides free or low-cost basic medical and hospital care. It's for citizens, permanent residents, and some temporary residents and is made up of the Medicare Benefits Schedule (MBS), Pharmaceutical Benefits Scheme (PBS), and Safety Nets.

Medicare covers doctor visits, medical tests, and public hospital stays, ensuring you don't bear the full financial burden. But... it doesn't extend to everything, like dental care (except specific cases), many allied health services, cosmetic surgeries, glasses, and hearing aids.

In a nutshell, Medicare is your healthcare hero, but it's not a one-size-fits-all. Remember what's in and what's out and that these can change.

"Medicare has saved me thousands of dollars throughout my life! I always took it for granted, but now I know how it works, I'm even more grateful."

MEDICARE BENEFITS SCHEME (MBS)

The MBS is like a giant net that's there to catch you when it comes to healthcare expenses.

The MBS is a very long list of medical services, procedures, and tests, each with a unique code. These codes matter when you see your doctor or specialist for your surgery. They decide how much Medicare chips in for your care. It's like a passcode, ensuring you're not left with the whole financial load. From check-ups to procedures, the MBS has your back, making sure your health doesn't drain your funds.

Here's how you can find out what's covered by the MBS:

01

MBS Online

You can look up procedures or item numbers yourself by typing in the service name or number. Then, you'll find out what's covered and Medicare's contribution. Easy peasy!

02

Medicare Cost Finder

This is similar to the MBS search function but more user-friendly, in my humble opinion.

03

Ask your Doctor or Their Staff

Your doctor and their staff are familiar with the MBS and can guide you on what services are covered for your surgery.

04

Speak to Medicare

If you're unsure about a particular service, you can always call Medicare's helpline on 13 20 11.

BULK BILLING

Bulk Billing is like a golden ticket for healthcare. When a doctor or specialist bulk bills, it means they accept the Medicare benefit as full payment for their services and a $0 payment from you.

So, if you're bulk billed, you won't have to pay anything out of your own pocket. For someone going in for major surgery, bulk billing can take a load off your mind, as your medical expenses are taken care of by Medicare.

 **TIP**: Search the **HealthDirect Service Finder** to find health professionals and services that Bulk Bill.

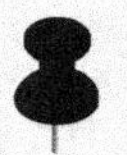 **NOTE:** Bulk billing doesn't cover all health professionals or services. You need to do research on what you're covered for based on your circumstances.

PARTIAL BILLING

This is when the doctor charges more than the Medicare benefit for their services. You'll need to pay the difference, known as the "gap". The Medicare benefit will still cover some of the cost, but you must contribute the rest. Some doctors choose to partially bill to reflect the actual cost of their services or to provide extra services beyond what Medicare covers.

MEDICARE SAFETY NET

The Medicare Safety Net is your backup for covering costs outside of the hospital.

> **NOTE:** The safety nets step in to help out when you've got hefty medical bills for stuff outside the hospital. Just remember, they won't kick in for things that aren't on the Medicare Benefits Schedule (MBS) or for MBS services done in a hospital.

When you hit a spending limit, the safety net kicks in to ease the load. Imagine facing piles of medical bills for your surgery because of extra blood tests or GP visits. Once you cross a certain point, the Safety Net steps in to cut your costs. No more feeling buried under bills—it's your safety cushion, keeping your finances steady.

The spending limit changes regularly. Here are some ways you can check the limit and how you're tracking against it.

01 **Medicare Express Plus App**

Get the app and click on 'Safety Net'.

02 **MyGov App**

Get the app and click on 'Medicare', then look for the Safety Net.

03 **Call Medicare - 132 011**

Have your Medicare Number handy and give them a bell.

PHARMACEUTICAL BENEFITS SCHEME (PBS)

The PBS is a healthcare hero who makes vital medicines affordable. It acts like a money-saving middleman between medicine makers and you. It gets the makers to agree on lower prices for several vital medications, which means you don't have to pay full price when you need them for your surgery or treatment.

A couple of things to remember:

01 Co-Payments

While the PBS reduces the cost of medications, you'll still need to make a contribution when you pick up your prescription.

02 Prescription Only

The PBS only covers medication that can be prescribed, it doesn't cover things like vitamins, supplements, or some over-the-counter medicines

03 Select Medicines Only

Not all medications are automatically included in the PBS. Medications must be approved and listed on the PBS Schedule to be subsidised. The Schedule is regularly updated to include new drugs and treatments.

Finding out if your meds are included on the PBS is as easy as pie! Ask your GP or Pharmacist about the medicines you've been or will be prescribed. Then, you can hop onto the official PBS website (https://www.pbs.gov.au) and type in the name of your medicine or its active ingredient. The website will tell you if it's a PBS superstar or not.

 **TIP**: If your prescribed medication isn't on the PBS, there might still be a way to access it affordably. Patient Access Programs can assist with medications not covered by the PBS, making them more accessible. Check with your healthcare provider or the pharmaceutical company to see if you qualify and how to apply.

PBS SAFETY NET

The PBS Safety Net kicks in when you've spent a certain amount on listed medicines in a calendar year. Each time you pick up a prescription from the pharmacy, your expenses are recorded under your Medicare number. So be sure to take your Medicare card with you every time. Once you hit the Safety Net threshold, your pharmacist will issue you a Safety Net Card, which ensures you receive discounted medicine prices for the rest of the calendar year.

Now, what if you're visiting different pharmacies for your medications? No worries – your expenses are still tracked if you use your Medicare card.

 **TIP**: If you forget to use your Medicare card, keep the receipts of your prescription medications and use them as evidence to make a claim

Here are some ways you can check how you're tracking for the Medicare Safety Net:

01 **Medicare Express Plus App**

Get the app and click on 'Safety Net'.

02 **MyGov App**

Get the app and click on 'Medicare'.

03 **Call PBS - 1800 020 613**

Have your Medicare Number and medication names handy.

TREATMENT PLANS

A Medicare Treatment Plan helps you manage your chronic condition with a coordinated care approach. Created by your GP, it outlines your healthcare needs and goals. It allows you to access subsidised treatments from various healthcare professionals, making your care more comprehensive and affordable.

Chat with your GP or Mental Health Professional to explore these plans. Here are two treatment plans that may help you prepare for surgery.

01 **Chronic Disease Treatment Plan**

This plan is your financial friend if you're dealing with ongoing health issues. Your GP collaborates with Specialists to create a game plan that prioritises your health and manages costs. It's a personalised roadmap guiding you toward effective treatments with less financial strain.

02 **Mental Health Care Treatment Plan**

For emotional well-being, this plan is your wallet-friendly ticket to prioritise mental wellness. It offers support and guidance without hefty bills. Subsidised sessions with mental health professionals provide help while minimising financial worry.

HOSPITALS

Hospitals are complicated, so there is a whole chapter about it coming up. But here is what you need to know in relation to money.

If you're admitted to a **public hospital**, Medicare covers a significant portion of your medical expenses. In essence, it should be free. This includes doctor's fees, diagnostic tests, and most medical services provided during your stay. Sometimes there may be some costs, which you should be told about beforehand.

During your stay in a **private hospital**, Medicare typically covers a portion of the fees. However, it's important to note that Medicare does not cover all the costs, and you'll need private health insurance and your own money to cover the costs.

Basically, Medicare works alongside both public and private hospitals to provide essential medical coverage.

Other Government Support

CONCESSION CARDS

You might qualify for special government concession cards that offer financial support. These cards are designed to assist those facing financial difficulties due to their health circumstances. Here are two key government concession cards:

01 **Health Care Card**

This card provides access to reduced-cost medical services and prescriptions. If you receive certain government benefits, such as JobSeeker Payment, Parenting Payment, or Disability Support Pension, you might be eligible. With this card, you'll get benefits like cheaper prescriptions, bulk-billed doctor visits, and lower costs for essentials like public transport.

02 **Low Income Health Care Card**

This card is for people with lower incomes who aren't receiving specific government payments. It provides similar benefits as the Health Care Card, helping you manage medical expenses more effectively.

Curious about your eligibility? Check out:
- Government websites, offices, and helplines
- Community organisations
- Financial counsellors
- Healthcare providers

Keep in mind that eligibility criteria can change, so stay updated with reliable sources. Exploring your eligibility could offer valuable financial assistance during your major surgery journey.

OTHER SUBSIDIES

If you need additional care or support due to your surgery, you might like to check out other government programs like the Disability Support Pension, Carer Payment, and Carer Allowance. Also, investigate the JobSeeker Payment or Parenting Payment if your ability to work is temporarily impacted. Additionally, explore the Family Tax Benefit, which provides financial help for families with dependent children.

Medical Travel Support

Navigating the journey of major surgery often involves not just the medical aspects but also the logistics of travel.

Luckily, all states and territories have some kind of Patient Assisted Travel Scheme (PATS) that will help cover things like transport and accommodation for you and a carer. Some PATS are more generous than others, and of course, the rules are all different.

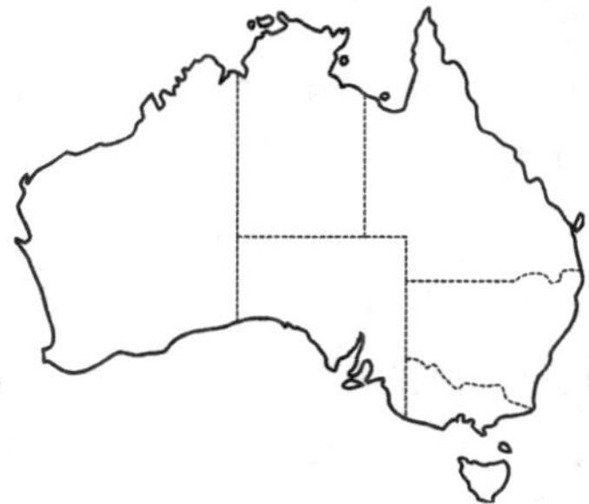

Check out details for your state or territory here:

- **Australian Capital Territory:** Interstate Patient Travel Assistance Scheme
- **Northern Territory:** Patient Assistance Travel Scheme
- **New South Wales:** Isolated Patients Travel and Accommodation Assistance Scheme
- **Queensland:** Patient Travel Subsidy Scheme
- **South Australia:** Patient Assistance Transport Scheme
- **Tasmania:** Patient Travel Assistance Scheme
- **Western Australia**: Patient Assisted Travel Scheme and Interstate Patient Travel Scheme
- **Victoria:** Victorian Patient Transport Assistance Scheme

Disability Parking Permit

Don't skip this bit thinking that disability parking permits are just for old folk. They aren't! These permits can be a game-changer for anyone, regardless of age, recovering from major surgery or not mobile before surgery.

These nifty permits give you closer parking spots, so you don't have to splurge on premium parking. Plus, they can help you cut down on transportation costs by making it easier to access essential places. And let's not forget, they're a lifesaver when it comes to conserving energy—a win-win for your well-being and your wallet.

To snag one, here's the scoop:
- First, check if you meet the eligibility criteria, which usually include having a severe and permanent disability or a temporary disability due to surgery.
- Next, get a medical certificate from your doctor to support your application.
- Then, complete the application form from your state or territory authority.

"I've have been using this Permit on and off since I was 20. It's made doing simple things like grocery shopping possible, and helped me stay social."

Private Health Insurance

Private health insurance is like an extra layer of protection for your health. You can choose to buy it in addition to the healthcare services the government provides through Medicare.

Private health insurance coverage for major surgery will vary depending on your policy type and the specific procedure you're undergoing.

WHAT'S IN

Generally, private health insurance MIGHT cover the following aspects of major surgery:
- Hospital Accommodation
- Theatre Fees
- Doctor's Fees
- Prostheses and Medical Devices (e.g. heart valve)
- In-Hospital Services
- Rehabilitation and Post-operative Care
- Ambulance Services

Some health insurers now include travel and accommodation under "Hospital Cover," so check that out.

WHAT'S OUT

It's important to note that private health insurance may not cover everything related to major surgery. Standard exclusions or limitations MAY include:

- Pre-Existing Conditions
- Out-of-Pocket Expenses
- Non-medical costs (e.g. travel and accommodation for surgery)
- Certain Treatments and Procedures
- Cosmetic Procedures

CHECKING YOUR COVERAGE

It's crucial to thoroughly review your private health insurance policy, including its coverage, exclusions, waiting periods, and benefit limits, before undergoing major surgery.

There are a few steps to find out what you're covered for.

01 **Review Policy Doc**

Check your policy and schedules for what's in and out. You can find policies in the email you got when you signed up or renewed your cover, or by logging into their online portal.

02 **Contact Insurer**

Give em' a call - have your Medicare Item Numbers and surgery deets handy. Ask questions and clarify coverage details with customer service.

03 **Talk to your financial counsellor**

Have a chat with your financial counsellor to work out what's covered.

Not sure what to say when you call them, try this:

Hello, I'm calling to understand what my private health insurance covers for major surgery. I have a [mention your policy name or number] policy with your company. I'm currently facing the prospect of undergoing major surgery and would like to know what aspects of the procedure are covered under my policy.

Could you please help me by answering a few questions?
- *I've been provided with these Medicare Items Number [xxx], are they covered?*
- *Do you have any recommended hospitals for my procedure? My specialist has recommended [xxx] hospital, is that included?*
- *What hospital and rehabilitation services does my policy cover, and what won't it cover?*
- *Does my hospital cover include travel and accommodation?*
- *Is there anything else I should be aware of?*

Thank you for your time and assistance. Could you please confirm our discussion in writing by emailing me the details.

Superannuation Insurance

Super funds come with insurance cover baked right in. This can be like having a hidden helper in your corner, ready to step in if you're facing a financial squeeze due to unexpected medical expenses or long-term leave from work.

Here's the scoop on the main types of insurance that can be tucked away in your super fund.

INCOME PROTECTION

This is like having a backup plan for your paycheck. If you're sidelined from work due to illness or injury, income protection insurance can provide regular financial support to keep your finances afloat during your recovery journey.

TRAUMA

Think of this as a helping hand in the face of severe medical conditions. If you're diagnosed with a critical illness like cancer or a heart attack, trauma insurance offers a financial lifeline with a lump sum payout. This can help you navigate the challenges that come with such a diagnosis.

TOTAL AND PERMANENT DISABILITY

Imagine this as a guardian angel for your income. If you're faced with a medical setback that prevents you from working permanently, TPD insurance steps in. It offers a payout to help with living costs, medical bills, and other essentials while you focus on your recovery.

LIFE

Think of this as a shield for your loved ones. If the unexpected occurs and you're no longer around, your beneficiaries could receive a lump sum payout from your super fund's life insurance. This can provide a safety net to cover expenses and secure their future when you're not there to do so.

CHECKCING YOUR COVERAGE

Similar to private health insurance, there are ways to seek assistance and ensure you make the most informed decisions about your insurance coverage. Here's how you can get help:

01   **Review Policy Doc**

Check your policy and schedules for what's in and out. You can find policies in the email you got when you signed up or renewed your cover or by logging into their online portal.

02 **Contact Your Super Fund**

Give em' a call - have your Super Fund and surgery details handy. Ask questions and clarify coverage details with customer service.

03 **Talk to your financial counsellor**

Have a chat with your financial counsellor to work out what's covered.

04 **Talk to Human Resources at your work**

If works in the mix, chat with your HR about insurance options.

Not sure what to say when you call them, try this:

Hello, I'm calling to understand what my super fund insurance covers for major surgery. I have a [mention your policy name or number] policy with your company. I'm currently facing the prospect of undergoing major surgery and would like to know if my situation is covered under my policy.

Thank you for your time and assistance. Could you please confirm our discussion in writing by sending me an email with the details.

EARLY ACCESS

You can dip into your retirement savings early for specific reasons, like medical treatment. It's called *early release of superannuation.*

Here's what you need to know:

01 **Get Financial Advice**

Before you decide, talk to your financial counsellor.

02 **Medical Reasons**

You *might* get early access if you need treatment not available through the public health system and it greatly affects your quality life.

03 **Apply to the ATO**

To ask for early release, submit a request to the Australian Taxation Office (ATO). They'll review it.

TIP: Remember, early access is a **serious choice** that impacts retirement savings. Chat with a Financial Counsellor to decide what's best for your future. Do your homework!

Crowd Funding

Over the years, people have found some pretty cool ways to raise cash to pay for expensive medical procedures, equipment or medications that the government or insurance just don't cover. The main one is Crowdfunding – basically, you set yourself up on an existing online platform, explain why you need cash, and then people just give it to you! How amazing is that! You can also host events to get donations.

With this one, just be sure to do some homework on the terms and conditions of the platform you're crowdfunding from and check the rules on if/how to pay tax on what you make from your crowd.

Charities

Over 600 charities are working in the health sector, ready to be your champion! They're like your support squad, ready to tackle medical costs, travel expenses, and daily life challenges while you recover. They can help you with cash for medical bills, cover travel costs, and even ensure you've got the basics like toothbrushes and snacks. If you're travelling for treatment, they have comfy places for you and your family to stay.

Here are some star-studded champs that can be your go-to support team:

- Heart Foundation
- HeartKids Australia
- Cancer Council Australia
- Rare Cancers Australia
- Lung Foundation Australia
- Endometriosis Australia
- Australian Red Cross
- Angel Flight Australia

Remember, each of these has its own way of doing things. So, contact them directly to get the lowdown on the support they offer and how to get it.

World Bank of Mum & Dad

"I'll admit that I dipped into the "World Bank of Mum & Dad" more than a few times in my twenties. Yep, I leaned on my parents when things got tough. And you know what? It's totally okay. Having that safety net is a privilege, and I'm seriously grateful for it. Thanks, mum and Dad xx"

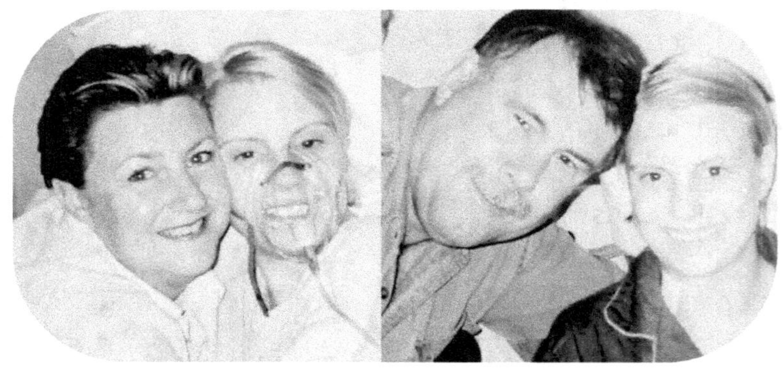

2004 - 21 Years Old - With Mum (Marion Roche) and Dad (Robert Pendrick) for My Fourth Open-Heart Surgery

Now, here's the deal for you. If your parents are in a position to lend a hand and you find yourself in a spot where you need help, don't let your pride stand in the way. Seriously, it's okay to ask for help. Your finances don't need to take a nosedive when there's a helping hand waiting for you.

House and Life Bills

If money's feeling a bit tight and you're juggling bills like gas, electricity, and your phone or even dealing with unexpected fines, talk to your Financial Counselor. You have options! The key is to be proactive. Kickstart the conversation early, especially before your surgery.

Here are some options you can talk to your financial counsellor or your provider about:

01 Mortgage and Rent

There might be options like pausing payments or securing a favourable deal.

02 Utilities

Options can include extending payment due dates, setting up instalment plans, or applying for rebates. Stay ahead to avoid service suspension and potential credit score impact.

Check out the **National Debt Helpline's** tips to get your bills under control: https://ndh.org.au/Debt-problems/Electricity-gas-and-water-bills/

03 Insurance Premiums

For insurance premiums on home, car, life, or health coverage, options could be tailored payment plans or temporary adjustments. If claiming, enquire about reducing or delaying excess payments.

04

Council Rates

Options may include instalment plans, payment delays, or interest write-offs.

Check out the **National Debt Helpline's** step-by-step guide to paying your rates: https://ndh.org.au/debt-problems/council-rates/

05

Strata Levies

Explore alternate payment arrangements.

06

Fines

Options might be extended payment times or utilising Centrelink deductions. Avoid repercussions like licence suspension or legal action.

TIP: Be proactive! Don't hesitate to utilise resources like your Financial Counsellor or the National Debt Helpline

School and Uni Fees

SCHOOL FEES

School fees and major surgery might seem like a tricky equation, but there's a playbook for this, too. Firstly, open up communication channels with your child's school or college. Believe it or not, they're often more understanding and flexible than you'd think. They might have options like deferred payment plans or scholarships that can give you a bit of breathing room. Some schools even have support programs for students going through tough times, like having parents go through medical procedures.

UNIVERSITY FEES AND DEBT

If you have HECS / HELP debt, you have options for paying it. Talk to your university's student services about your situation—they're wizards at finding solutions. They might have options like deferring your payments or providing you with some extra support during this time.

Hospital Add-on Costs

There are always sneaky costs that might pop up when going in for surgery.

Keep a stash of money to cover things like:

01 Parking

While hospitals are all about healing, parking fees can be a bit of a pain.

02 Travel Costs

If you're traveling to the hospital, petrol costs can add up.

03 Accommodation

Your loved ones might need a place to crash while you're in the hospital.

04 Food

Hospital food isn't exactly like dining out. So, budget for some snacks or meals during your stay.

05 Incidentals

Those little expenses that might catch you by surprise.

 **TIP**: Don't forget change for the lolly trolly - you can get magazines, food, toys and more

Budgeting

Wohoo - you made it to the end of the heftiest chapter!

Way to go!!

 **ACTION STEP:**
Map out your surgery budget

"I don't want anyone to ever struggle with money and surgery like I have. I know budgeting and money are not people's favourite topics. But, there is so much I wish someone would have told me about money and surgery! Enough to fill a hefty chapter, you might say."

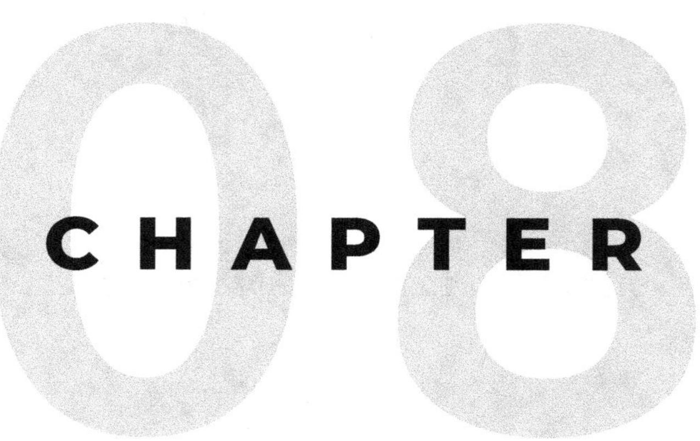

CHAPTER

Hospitals

"We are so lucky in Australia to have such amazing hospitals!"

The question of whether to go to a public or private hospital is a personal one.

I won't tell you which one to choose here. I'll just give you information and some questions to ask to make your own decision.

Public Hospitals

When it comes to how our public hospital system operates, well, it's complicated. Imagine it like divorced parents having shared custody over the kids – one parent is the federal government, the other parent is the state/territory governments, and the kids are the hospitals. Both parents want what's best for the kids but come at it from different viewpoints. The feds have slightly different arrangements with each ex (state/territory government), so the kids share some of the same toys, but some have cooler stuff than others. It all comes down to what's negotiated in the settlement!

The federal government sets national hospital policies and regulates the system, while the Independent Health and Aged Care Pricing Authority (IHACPI) determines the needed funds. They gather data from hospitals and decide how much to allocate. State/territory governments also contribute funds and manage the day-to-day operations of public hospitals in their regions. They ensure quality and safety.

For those of you with private health insurance, some policies even have special agreements with certain public hospitals, offering exclusive perks for specific treatments.

When it comes to public hospitals, there are a few things to remember:

01   **Access**

If you have a Medicare card, you can access public hospitals regardless of your ability to pay.

02 Wait Times

Sometimes, there might be queues for planned visits or specialist appointments.

03 Services

While public hospitals are great, they might not offer all the luxuries or specialised services you want.

04 Doctors

You'll likely be assigned a relevant doctor for your condition with no choice.

05 Costs

It's Free! But some extras, like TV, specific foods, or certain services, might cost money.

Private Hospitals

Welcome to the world of Australian private hospitals – where you're the star, and healthcare excellence takes centre stage! Imagine being able to tailor your hospital visit to your preferences. Choose your dream team of specialists and enjoy fast-tracked care without long wait times.

While you don't need private health insurance to use a private hospital, having it will cover more costs. Medicare can still help cover some medical services in private hospitals, so you're not alone.

Private health insurers form agreements with specific hospitals to expand their policyholders' access to healthcare. These agreements, called hospital agreements, provide policyholders with a broader choice of medical services at these preferred hospitals while helping insurers control costs and maintain quality care standards.

In summary, here are the 6 things you need to know:

01 **Expertise Matters**

Check the hospital's success with your specific surgery. A proven track record and skilled surgeons are critical.

02 **Quality Counts**

Look for top-notch care. Consider patient reviews, accreditation, and safety measures.

03 Facilities

Assess amenities and comforts for your recovery, like private rooms and advanced tech.

04 Specialist Team

Ensure access to a range of specialists for comprehensive care from start to finish.

05 Insurance Insights

Know your coverage. Confirm that the hospital and procedure of your choice are covered.

06 Cost

Your private insurance will cover some, but you'll likely have to pay some money from your own pocket. Do the calculations and talk to the hospital.

Your Choice

Choosing between private and public healthcare is a big decision. Here's a quick guide to help you choose what's best for you:

01 Budget

Figure out what you can afford. Private care will cost more, while public care is free (or has small fees).

02 Health Needs

If you need a particular type of surgery that is only done at a select few hospitals (like transplants) or your specialists recommend a particular hospital, then your options are more limited.

03 Insurance Cover

If you have private health insurance, your insurer may have agreements with particular hospitals, and it may depend on your policy coverage.

04 Waiting Times

Public hospitals might mean longer waits, while private care can be faster and more predictable.

05 Control

You'll have more control and choices in private care. In public care, you'll likely have less control but still good care.

06 Hospital Reputation

Research the quality of hospitals near you – private and

06

public. They may have particular reputations to be aware of.

07

Family Needs

If you have a family or are caring for a child having surgery there are factors to consider to best accommodate everyones needs.

08

Luxury v Basics

Private care has perks like private rooms. If you value comfort, it's worth considering.

09

Surgeon Availability

Some surgeons only operate in public and private hospitals; others operate out of just one. If the surgeon only operates out of one hospital type, this will limit your choice.

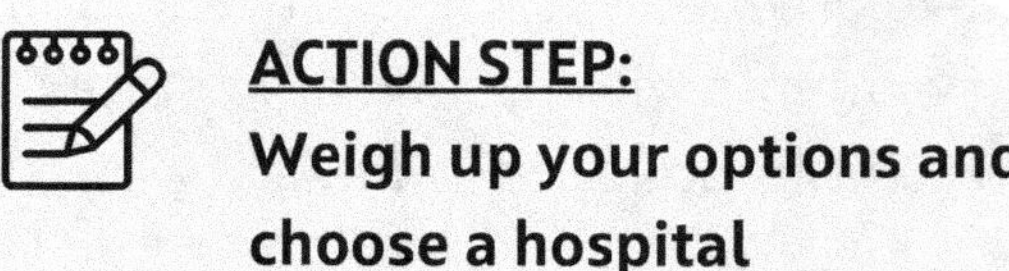

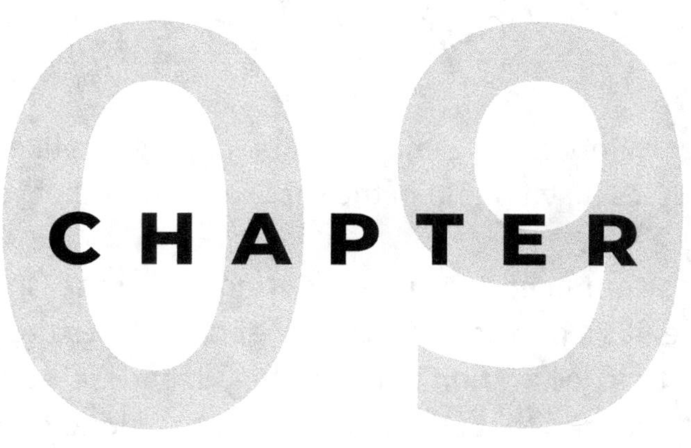

"There is such a thing as work-life-surgery balance!"

Navigating the work-life-surgery tightrope is tricky, but there are heaps of ways to ease the load. This chapter is here to guide you through the uncertainty, to be a reassuring voice in the midst of confusion.

 **NOTE:** This chapter does not include legal or professional workplace advice. Please consider your situation, seek professional advice and do your homework.

Work Mindset

Your career is important. Major surgery might seem like it might derail it, but it's just a bump in the road, not the end of your career.

Recognising your need for support during this phase isn't just a smart move–it's a powerful decision that challenges the notion of weakness. It's a declaration that your health and well-being are non-negotiable and that taking a moment to tend to them isn't a misstep–it's a statement of strength.

To give you some inspiration, here are some people who have stepped away from their careers for a little while for health reasons and have continued on to great things:

- Selena Gomez - Singer/Actor – Kidney Transplant
- Hayley Raso – Matilda's Player – Broke her back and came back to play in the 2023 FIFA World Cup and the 2024 Olympics
- Kevin Rudd – Aussie Prime Minister, now Ambassador to the USA – had open heart surgery in between jobs

"I've also had to take time out of my career on many occasions for things like major surgery, long COVID, and just life with chronic illness. I still managed to scale the corporate ladder, earn six figures, manage a team, and start my own business! If I can do it, so can you!"

Working out Leave

Have a heart-to-heart (pun intended!) with your surgeon and medical crew about the nitty-gritty of your job. Walk them through your typical workday, from your daily commute to punching out. Ask your doctor for their insights on how much time off you might require. Each situation is as unique as a fingerprint, and your leave plan will be crafted to fit the type of surgery you're facing and what's most practical for you.

In many hospitals, your surgery date may not be set until a week or so before, and even then, it might change on the day. This can make it tricky to negotiate your leave. Don't for a second feel guilty about stuffing your around boss about it. The date of your surgery is usually well out of your control. Yes, it can make for some awkward conversations, but there is not much you can do about how the hospital system works.

Finding out you need major surgery is a big deal; adding the uncertainty of when and how much leave you'll need can feel like a double whammy. Sometimes, it can be more than you anticipated as well, so take a deep breath; it's completely normal. This is where your mental health toolkit comes into play. Go unpack your feelings with your mental health professional and use those tools you've built up.

Your medical team might also tell you that predicting your exact leave duration is a bit like guessing the length of a piece of string – they can't be 100% sure. Your response to surgery and recovery will be unique. While the time spent in the hospital post-op is typically fixed (all going to plan), the recovery journey can vary between people.

So, you'll have to navigate this a bit on the fly, which can be tricky when dealing with your boss. However, there are strategies to help you manage this situation in a way that benefits you and your workplace.

"Prepping for my fifth open heart surgery, I was at the peak of my career – earning great money, jet-setting around the world, and rubbing shoulders with the big shots. I had poured blood, sweat, and tears into that job. But when I realised, I needed 6-8 weeks of leave, it was a curveball in my dream job. I made the tough decision to step back temporarily to relieve the pressure. About three months post-op, I was able to return to my dream job and continue my career journey."

Disability Discrimination

According to the Disability Discrimination Act 1992 (DDA), when you're dealing with medical stuff in the workplace, you might fall under the "disabled" category. This can be confusing as you may not classify as disabled to get access to government subsidies (e.g. disability payments) or feel like you are, but you may well be in the workforce.

The DDA ensures that no one can discriminate against you based on medical conditions and surgery. It also ensures that you make the choice of whether to disclose your medical condition to the boss. However, in some cases, workplaces may need to be aware of a medical condition if it affects your ability to do your job safely. Telling the boss can be necessary to assess reasonable changes.

It's illegal for you to be discriminated against due to your medical condition or upcoming surgery at work. Discrimination can look like:
- Blocking your leave
- Demoting you (forcing you to take a more junior role)
- Denying you a promotion, transfer or opportunities
- Messing with the terms and conditions of your employment (like your pay rate, work hours, and leave)
- Firing or sacking you
- Bullying, harassing or excluding you

Your workplace is legally bound to support making "reasonable" changes to help you work before and after surgery. Think of things like flexible hours, easing back into work, or getting some special gear. But what's "reasonable" can be up for debate; they might be within their rights to say nah, which you can contest.

 **TIP**: Check out more about the Disability Discrimination Act 1992, including what the exclusions are here: https://humanrights.gov.au/our-work/disability-rights/disability-discrimination

 **TIP**: Check out **Job Access** for more details of your rights and responsibilities and general help https://www.jobaccess.gov.au/

"After 5 open heart surgeries, it never occurred to me that I was disabled during the surgery process... even when I had a disability parking permit. The term disability has a bit of baggage, so I've worked through it with my counsellor and am now proud to say that I have a disability. If this is a big mental shift for you, take the time to process it. Own it as the temporary or permanent badge of honour it is".

Advocacy

When you're facing major surgery and work responsibilities, your voice becomes your strongest asset. Advocacy means confidently expressing your needs, concerns, and aspirations and ensuring they're heard and addressed.

Whether discussing leave options, negotiating a phased return to work, or seeking reasonable accommodations, your proactive stance demonstrates your commitment to your well-being and professional growth.

Remember, no one knows your journey better than you do, and advocating for yourself ensures that your needs are considered, your rights are upheld, and your potential is recognised.

Leave Entitlements

Leave entitlements are important rules set out in the Fair Work Act that say you can take a break from work when you're having major surgery and will not lose your job. These rules ensure you have the chance to heal and get better without worrying about work.

There are a few different types of leave you can use while you're away from work. These depend on your industry, awards, and employment type. Do your homework on these!

Here is a summary of the basics.

SICK (AKA PERSONAL) LEAVE

With paid sick leave by your side, you can focus on your recovery without worrying about your paycheck taking a hit. If you're employed full-time or part-time, you can take paid sick leave for surgery (cha-ching!). You get 10 paid sick days per year if you're full-time and a proportion of that if you're part-time. Things are a bit different if you're employed casually. You won't be entitled to paid sick leave, but you can get unpaid leave.

UNPAID LEAVE

Unpaid leave is the wildcard in your arsenal. While it might not come with a paycheck, unpaid leave ensures your job remains untouched while you give your undivided attention to your health.

ANNUAL (AKA HOLIDAY) LEAVE

While usually reserved for holidays, annual leave can also be used for medical needs. It lets you dive into recovery mode while enjoying the perks of paid time away. Yes, its annoying to have to use it for something other than a holiday, but it sure beats not being paid.

LONG SERVICE LEAVE

The reward for your dedication and loyalty. Long service leave offers you an extended period of paid time off, perfect for those who've been working side by side with their employers for years.

BONUS LEAVE

Workplaces sometimes offer additional leave options, such as compassionate leave, for unforeseen situations. This offers even more flexibility as you navigate your way back to health.

FINDING OUT YOUR LEAVE

To know exactly what you're entitled to, you can:
- look at your work contract, Award, Enterprise Agreement or intranet

- have a chat with your boss
- chat to someone in the human resources department at your workplace
- Use the Fair Work Ombudsman Leave Calculator (https://calculate.fairwork.gov.au/leave)
- Check out this handy video about leave from the Fair Work Ombudsman: https://www.fairwork.gov.au/leave/sick-and-carers-leave

You gotta let your boss know as soon as possible that you'll need the leave and how long you think it will be for. You'll also need to show the boss evidence that you're having the surgery (or that the leave is for medical purposes). You can do this through a medical certificate or statutory declaration. Each workplace can have its own agreement on what steps you need to go through, when, and what evidence you'll need, so do some research.

Mix n' Match

Think of your leave options as puzzle pieces, each fitting together to create the leave and support you need. Mixing and matching these leave types lets you design a recovery plan that's as unique as your journey. Combine sick leave with unpaid leave for an extended healing period, or tap into your accrued annual leave for a seamless transition to recovery mode. It's up to you and the boss to work it out.

Also, think about how your mix-and-match goes with your Budget plan. You might need to combine government subsidies, insurance, charity support, and the World Bank of Mum and Dad with your leave entitlements to get you through.

"I've found that mixing and matching my leave has worked really well for me and my employers over the years".

ACTION STEP:
What are your leave entitlements?

ACTION STEP:
How are you going to mix n' match your leave and align it with your budget?

Returning to Work

After getting through the surgery, the path back to the workplace might require some strategic navigation. Here are some ways to achieve the right work-life-recovery balance.

PHASED RETURN TO WORK

A phased return to work is like having a bridge that spans your healing time and your return to work responsibilities. With a phased return, you don't wholly dive back into the hustle and bustle of work. Instead, you gradually ease into your work hours and tasks over a set timeframe. This approach is all about flexibility and finding what suits you and your employer best.

You might kick things off with reduced working hours and build back up slowly. This could look like three half days for two weeks, then three full days, and then a whole five-day work week. Or you could start working from home for a portion of the week and slowly build up to being in the office or on-site. It could even mean taking on tasks that are less demanding physically or mentally at first. It's about listening to your unique needs and tailoring your return to work to bring out the best in you.

REMOTE WORK
(AKA WORKING FROM HOME)

Remote work offers the chance to carry out your tasks from the sanctuary of your home, allowing for much-needed breaks and even a nap to recharge. This post-surgery perk provides a flexible way to keep work rolling while tending to medical appointments and your healing process, whether you're diving into tasks for a single day or developing a schedule that spans a few days a week.

FLEXIBLE ARRANGEMENTS

Think of flexible arrangements as the opportunity to paint your ideal work schedule. This can include adjusted start and finish times, compressed workweeks, job sharing, or working from home. After surgery, these arrangements can provide the space you need for follow-up appointments, treatments, or simply adjusting to your post-surgery routine.

"I've used each of these approaches over the years and adapt them for my workplace and how I'm feeling".

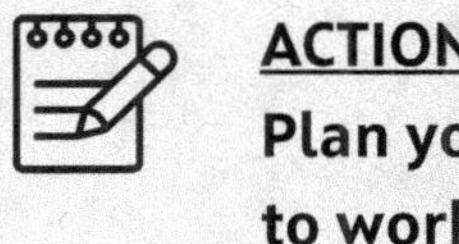
ACTION STEP:
**Plan your return
to work strategy**

Negotiating with the Boss

Your Boss can be your advocate, understanding your needs and providing the necessary support to ensure your work-life-surgery balance remains intact.

Chatting with "The Boss" can be a win-win situation. Sharing your surgery plans, recovery timeline, and any adjustments you might require lays the groundwork for a smooth journey ahead. It's about building trust between work and well-being.

NAVIGATING THE CONVERSATION

Approaching your boss to discuss taking leave for your upcoming surgery might seem daunting, but with a well-crafted plan, you can foster understanding and ensure a smoother journey.

A few things you might want to let the boss know:

01 **Dates**
What is the proposed start date of your leave and the duration.

02 **Medical Recommendations**
How long has your medical team recommended you have leave for and why.

03 **Type of Leave**

What type/s of leave do you recommend based on your research and allowances.

04 **Potential changes**

Note that things might change, like timings of the surgery (leave start date) and recovery (return date).

05 **Notifying others**

If you approve of them letting others in the workplace know your situation or not.

Not sure how to kick it off? Here's a guide of what you could say:

Hello [Boss's Name],

I wanted to have an open conversation with you regarding an important matter. I've recently learned that I need to undergo major surgery. This will likely include a range of medical appointments over time as well. While I understand the importance of my role at [Company Name], my well-being is also a priority.

I've been researching the leave policies and believe that we can create a plan that allows me to address my health needs within existing provisions. I would like to discuss the possibility of using a combination of [xxx] leave and [xxx] leave to ensure I have the time required for a successful recovery and can attend critical appointments. However, this may need to change, pending factors like my response to surgery and recovery and the speed of the healthcare system.

I value the work I do here and want to ensure a seamless

transition during my absence. I'm committed to making this process as smooth as possible, including planning ahead, providing updates when available, and handing over work for my time off. However, I understand that plans may change as I navigate the healthcare system, and I will do my best to keep you informed if this happens.

When it's convenient for you, I'd appreciate the opportunity to discuss this further. Your insights and guidance would be invaluable as I navigate this journey.

Thank you for your understanding, and I look forward to your response.

Best regards,
[Your Name]

This is just a template. Feel free to personalise it based on your relationship with your boss and your specific circumstances. The trick is to convey your need for leave in a professional and considerate manner, emphasising your commitment to both your health and your role within the company.

10 WAYS TO BOOST YOUR CHAT

01 Medical Certificates

Obtain a medical certificate from your healthcare provider detailing that you are having surgery and the recommended recovery period. This official document is your anchor, lending credibility to your request and

01 demonstrating your commitment to responsible planning.

02

Dress rehearsal

Practice what you're going to say with your support crew. Have some notes ready for when you meet your boss to ensure you cover all the important points.

03

Highlight Flexibility

Emphasise your flexibility in planning your leave. Discuss how you're open to adjusting your workload before and after your surgery, showing your commitment to maintaining your professional responsibilities where possible. (But make your health the priority).

04

Timely and Transparent Communication

Initiate the conversation well in advance, allowing ample time for your boss to adjust schedules and plan for your absence. Maintain open communication throughout the process to provide updates and address any concerns.

05

Written agreements

Pop what you both agree to in writing, noting that adjustments might need to be made depending on how your surgery journey and recovery go.

06

Changes Ahoy

Clearly explain that navigating the healthcare system isn't an exact science, so the leave needed can't be hard and fast. Many of the impacts of the surgery and your recovery will depend on factors like your response to the surgery, side effects, recovery response, and more. The leave you negotiate up front might need to be changed.

07 Address Potential Benefits

If applicable, discuss how your recovery period might offer insights or an opportunity to refine processes that could positively impact the team upon your return.

08 Reiterate Commitment

Emphasise your commitment to your role and the company's success. Assure your boss that you're focused on returning to peak condition and contributing effectively.

09 Highlight Your Track Record

If you have a history of reliability and dedication, remind your boss of your past contributions to the team. This demonstrates your value and willingness to go the extra mile.

10 Mental Load

Show you are being proactive in managing the mental load of work and major surgery by seeing a mental health professional, whether through the workplace EAP or any other method.

Remember, the key is to approach the conversation professionally and considerately. By arming yourself with evidence of medical necessity, a well-thought-out coverage plan, and a commitment to a smooth transition, you're setting the stage for a productive discussion that showcases your responsible approach to your health and professional obligations.

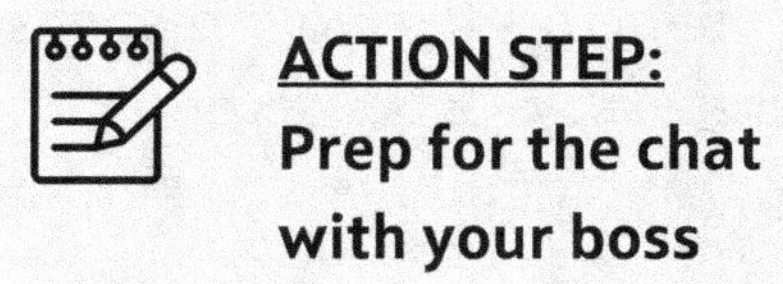

Where to get extra help

Confronting an unsupportive workplace atmosphere while preparing for surgery can cast a shadow on even the most determined spirits. Yet, even in the face of this adversity, you can steer the ship towards a more respectful and accommodating direction.

9 WAYS TO GET HELP AT WORK

01 **Know your ground**

Knowledge stands as your anchor amidst the confusion. Dive into your workplace policies, the Fair Work Act, and the Disability Discrimination Act. You can refer to these in discussions with your boss.

02 **Visit HR**

Proactively engage in a conversation with your Human Resources department about your concerns and experiences. HR is a source of guidance, equipped to clarify company policies and contribute to a more harmonious work environment.

03 **Document the Journey, Not the Drama**

As you navigate this, maintain a detailed account of conversations, emails, and any discrimination you've encountered. These records are critical in finding a resolution should the need arise.

Speak Out, with Steadiness

04

If you're prepared, address the issue directly with your Boss. Communicate calmly and confidently, underscoring your dedication to your role and the aim for a cooperative workspace.

Job Access

05

You can contact Job Access to get details about your rights and responsibilities. They also have very handy toolkits for your boss if they need some tips on managing your needs around the surgery.

Fair Work Ombudsman

06

Check out the Fair Work Ombudsman website for advice on how to address workplace issues.

Legal adviser

07

Contact a solicitor or a community legal centre whenever it suits you. They can help you out with various things, like drafting a formal demand letter. To find a solicitor, check out the law institute or law society in your state or territory, or find a community legal centre via https://clcs.org.au/.

Unions

08

For union members, they are ready to help you. Unions offer collective advocacy, amplifying your voice and striving for resolutions that align with your rights.

EAP

09

Your emotional well-being remains paramount in this challenging situation. Employee Assistance Programs offer confidential counsel, providing a safe space to feel heard, build confidence, and bolster your mindset.

You could also be a bit cheeky and give them this book. By skimming the content pages, they might learn everything you are juggling and improve their behaviour.

Navigating a hostile workplace environment can be emotionally draining. Seek solace from friends, family, or your mental health professional as you endure these challenges, striving for an environment that respects your rights and well-being.

Tech Support

"I wish I had access to even a quarter of the technology to support me through surgery that we have now."

In today's digital age, technology offers a massive helping hand in various aspects of our lives, and preparing for major surgery is no exception! From staying organised to accessing vital information, here are some ingenious ways to leverage tech.

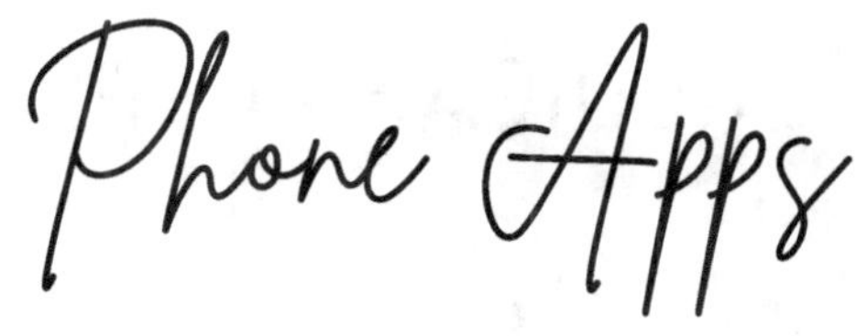

DIGITAL PAPERWORK APPS

There are many apps available now that can keep all your medical paperwork, like certificates, a description of your health condition by your doctor, or the need for particular medications. These help you stay in control and ensure you always have your paperwork.

To find the right app for you:
- Research Online: Seek popular medical document apps through reviews and forums.
- App Stores: Explore platforms like Apple App Store or Google Play for user insights.
- Ask a Healthcare Provider: Get app recommendations from your provider.
- Online Forums: Ask health communities like the Surgery Squad.
- Charities: Search out ones that have designed cool apps (like UpBeat by HeartKids)

MEDICATION TRACKING APPS

After surgery, you might have new medication routines to manage. Digital medication apps help track dosages, schedules, and set reminders—they're your virtual assistant for never missing a dose. Find the right app by using the same steps as for paperwork apps.

MEDICARE APP

Navigating the world of healthcare services is made simpler and more efficient with the Medicare app. This app puts the power of managing your healthcare benefits and services at your fingertips. You can also link your bank account directly to your Medicare account so benefits can be paid straight into it. No more paperwork or waiting in lines – you can conveniently access your Medicare details, submit claims, and keep track of benefits, all from the comfort of your smartphone.

HOSPITAL APPS

Some hospitals now have their own apps. That's very cool! You can download the app and fill out and submit all your paperwork digitally, get notifications of appointments, and even get records of your discussions with specialists. Contact your hospital to see if they have an app.

EMERGENCY CONTACTS IN PHONES

Add your medical history and emergency contact details to your phone. It's super easy to do and will be a huge help to people trying to help you in an emergency.

Digital Care

TELEHEALTH SERVICES

No more commutes or waiting rooms. Telehealth lets you easily arrange virtual consultations, transforming your home into a medical haven. Telehealth keeps germs at bay, reducing infection risk, and it can be cheaper than a face-to-face consult. Contact your health professional to see if you can connect via telehealth.

ELECTRONIC PRESCRIPTIONS

With electronic prescriptions, your doctor sends your prescription directly to your chosen pharmacy, phone number or email address, ensuring accuracy and reducing the risk of lost or misplaced prescriptions.

You can access your prescription details from your device of choice, whether it's your smartphone, tablet, or computer. This allows you to manage your medications effortlessly. Refills become seamless, with pharmacies keeping track and having your medication ready when needed.

Certain pharmacies also now have their own apps where you can order script refills and then just pop in to pick them up—no waiting in line. You can ask your pharmacist about this.

MY HEALTH RECORD

My Health Record is handy and innovative. It allows you to access and manage your health information in one centralised location. Keep track of prescriptions, test results, and medical history, ensuring you have a comprehensive overview of your health. My Health Record empowers you to share your information with healthcare professionals, streamlining the communication process and ensuring that your care is tailored to your unique needs.

While participation is voluntary (you can opt-out), the benefits of having a complete and accessible record of your health cannot be overstated.

HOME REHAB

Digital rehab programs offer a range of exercises designed to strengthen muscles, improve flexibility, and get your body back in action. However, it's essential to have a knowledgeable guide. Before you dive into these programs, please make sure you consult your healthcare provider. They can tailor the digital routines to your needs and ensure you're on the right track.

Medical Devices

HOME MEDICAL DEVICES

Elevate your self-care with home medical devices that shift the power of health management into your hands. From a blood pressure machine to a diabetes checker, these devices offer a personalised approach to well-being. Equip yourself with tools like pulse oximeters for oxygen level monitoring, thermometers for temperature checks, and scales for tracking weight and body composition.

With these devices, you're not just monitoring your health but actively participating in it. Take control of your wellness journey, armed with the knowledge and tools to make proactive choices for a healthier and more empowered life.

NOTE: Check with your Doctors if you need these devices before buying them.

Note: The quality of these devices can vary, so be sure to do your homework and speak to your Doctor and Pharmacist.

Note: Remember that home medical devices are support players, not stars. If you notice trends or abnormal results, make notes and speak to your doctor about them.

Digital Support

SMART DEVICES

Embrace the future of healthcare with smart watches and rings, wearable marvels that can become your health BFF. These sleek devices pack powerful features to monitor your well-being seamlessly. From tracking heart rate and sleep patterns to measuring activity levels and stress, they offer insights that empower you to take charge of your health. Get real-time updates on your vitals, set personalised fitness goals, and even receive gentle reminders to move or breathe.

CORDLESS HEADPHONES

Post-surgery recovery is demanding physically and mentally. This is where cordless headphones work their magic. While recovering post-surgery, surrounded by tubes and wires, adding headphone cords can add to the overwhelm. Cordless headphones offer an escape from the chaos, letting you enjoy music, podcasts, and relaxation apps without being connected to more cords.

"Cordless headphones have been an absolute game changer for me. I have many memories of being tangled in tubes and wires in the hospital, and getting tangled in headphone cords anytime would quickly bring back those memories. Cordless headphones make them feel like a treat, not a hospital device."

ENTERTAINMENT

Bring a world of entertainment and distraction to your hospital stay and recovery with your trusted devices. Whether it's a tablet, smartphone, or e-reader, these digital companions can transform your experience. Dive into captivating e-books, binge-watch your favourite shows, or listen to soothing meditation apps.

VIRTUAL ASSISTANTS

Meet Siri, Google Assistant, and Alexa – your digital concierge. Beyond answering questions and playing music, they manage tasks, appointments, and reminders. With a voice command, set medication alerts, send messages, and organise your to-do list.

DIGITAL COMMUNITY GROUPS

Many Facebook chat groups can be fantastic! They provide a safe, moderated space to talk about your surgery and support others. You can sit in the comfort of your home and have a whole cheer squad in the palm of your hand.

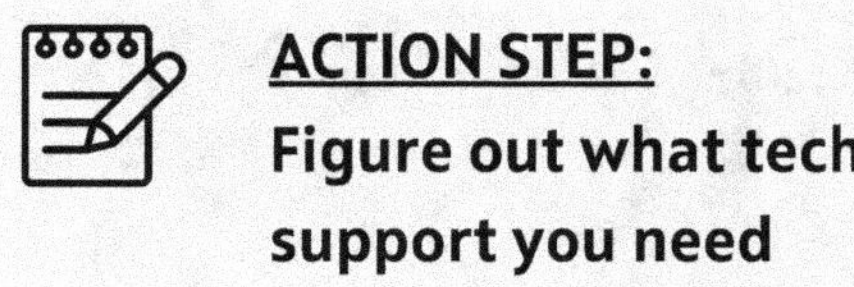

CHAPTER 11

Match Fit

While the exact surgery you'll be facing is unique to your situation, there are plenty of ways to prepare yourself physically to ensure you're ready for whatever challenges come your way. Think of it as getting ready for a big game – by honing your skills and building your strength, you'll be equipped to tackle anything that comes your way.

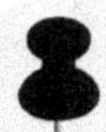 **NOTE:** Before you prepare for surgery, remember that your village–your medical team and support network–are your best guides on this journey.

Staying Active

Physical activity plays a vital role in getting you match-fit for your upcoming surgery. It's not about becoming an athlete overnight but rather finding activities that suit your current fitness level. Walking, swimming, or gentle yoga are options to consider. Regular movement helps improve overall strength, flexibility, and stamina, which can contribute to a smoother recovery process. Consult your healthcare team to determine your best activity plan based on your medical condition and goals.

PRACTICE MAKES PERFECT

Just like athletes train for the big game, you can prepare for your surgery by practising movements that will help you during your recovery. Whether you practice the right way to get out of a chair or bed, do gentle stretches, or even just take short walks, every bit of practice counts. Don't worry if it feels a little awkward at first—the more you practice, the more confident and prepared you'll become.

"After open heart surgery, taking care of your upper body is super important because your sternum needs time to heal. One cool trick is to practice getting in and out of chairs without pushing down on your hands, arms, or elbows – use your legs and core muscles instead. It might feel a bit weird at

Healthy Weight

Achieving and maintaining a healthy weight that aligns with your body's needs can significantly impact your surgical outcome. It can help reduce the risk of complications and promote better wound healing. Your healthcare team can guide you in achieving a healthy weight through nutrition and regular physical activity tailored to your circumstances.

HEALTHY WEIGHT HELPERS

01

Heart Foundation

Offers healthy eating guidelines and recipies.

02

CSIRO Total Wellbeing Diet

Offers Australia's most popular diet.

03

Delivery Options

There are loads of healthy eating options available that can be delivered straight to your door, like Light n Easy.

TIP: If your Doctors have recommended you lose weight for the surgery they should also be able to suggest ways to do this. Your pharmacist can also help.

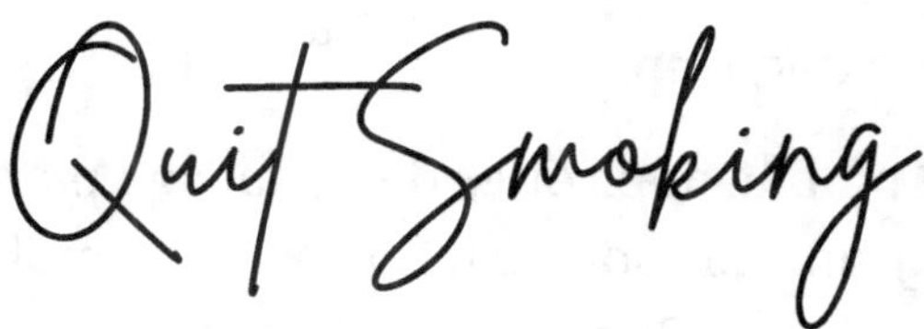

By quitting smoking (and vaping), you're giving your body the best chance for a successful surgery and smoother recovery. Facing major surgery while trying to quit smoking can be challenging. On one hand, quitting smoking before surgery can significantly improve your body's ability to heal, reduce the risk of complications, and enhance overall recovery. On the other hand, the stress and anxiety associated with surgery might make the urge to smoke even stronger.

It's a tricky balancing act, but your healthcare team is there to support you. They can guide you on the best approach to quitting.

RESOURCES FOR QUITTING SMOKING

01 **Quitline**

The Quitline is a free and confidential telephone counselling service that offers personalised advice and support to help you quit smoking. You can call 13 QUIT (13 78 48) to find out more.

02 **iCanQuit**

iCanQuit is an online platform that provides information, tools, and resources to help you quit smoking. Their website is www.icanquit.com.au, where you can find helpful tips, stories from other quitters, and a community of support.

03   Quit Smoking Apps

Several mobile apps offer personalised plans, progress tracking, and support to help you quit smoking. Examples include "My QuitBuddy" and "Quit for You - Quit for Two" for those who are pregnant.

04   Local Support Groups

Many communities offer local support groups or workshops for people who want to quit smoking. You can find them by doing a quick Google search.

05   Pharmacotherapy

Nicotine replacement therapies (NRT) are available over the counter at pharmacies. Have a chat with your pharmacist first.

06   GP or Healthcare Provider

Your GP can offer guidance on quitting smoking and may recommend suitable strategies or medications based on your individual needs. Be sure to ask if they will interact with your surgery or medication!

07   Public Health Programs

Some states in Australia have public health initiatives that provide resources and support for quitting smoking. Check with your local health department to see what programs are available in your area.

Your dedication to quitting is a significant step towards better health, both during and after your surgery.

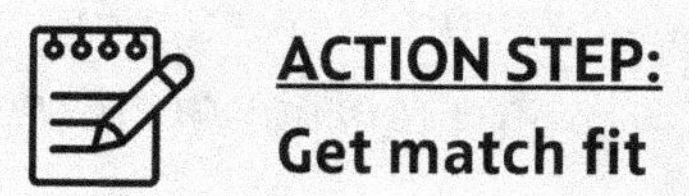

ACTION STEP:
Get match fit

CHAPTER 12

Women's Business

This section is designed exclusively for the incredible women having major surgery. Life's twists and turns often lead us to unexpected challenges, and facing surgery head-on can be empowering and overwhelming. In this section, I'm here to offer guidance and shine a light on the unique considerations that women may encounter.

Reproductive Health

Before you have surgery, it's wise to openly discuss your precious reproductive organs with your medical village. Let them know if there's anything that needs spotlighting—they're here to ensure your well-being and keep your reproductive health in order.

CONTRACEPTION

If you've got a contraception routine like a well-choreographed dance, it's essential to assess its compatibility with your upcoming surgery. Have a yarn with your medical village (including your pharmacist) to explore whether your chosen method will remain effective.

Some surgeries might play a bit of "hide and seek" with your contraceptive effectiveness, so it's best to always be prepared! Mix 'n' match with your medical team to find the ideal contraception that dances harmoniously with your surgery plan. Whether it's the Pill, the Patch, the Ring, the Rod or an army of barrier methods, keeping your reproductive organs safe is a top priority.

"Use some extra protection until you know for sure that your contraception meds aren't being diminished by pain meds or just the surgery recovery in general."

PERIODS

Major surgery can sometimes play a little prank on our menstrual rhythm, leaving our monthly visitor in a state of bewilderment. It's like your period's favourite rollercoaster ride got a surprise loop-de-loop.

So, don't be surprised if Aunt Flo decides to take a vacation, show up unexpectedly, or even party longer than usual. Your body might just be caught up in its own surgery sequel, and that's okay! Whether your period goes on a mini-vacay or decides to be the star of the show.

"My contraception had been working brilliantly until about six weeks post-op when my periods went haywire. The frequency of the periods was making me anaemic, so I had to change contraception. I'm not sure how open-heart surgery and periods are connected, but they were for me."

It's not unheard of to get a period while in hospital post-op. It might feel like the universe is playing a cosmic joke on you, but trust me, you're not alone if this happens to you. The hospital staff are seasoned experts who've seen every twist, turn, and unexpected guest appearance. Seriously, they've witnessed it all, and your surprise visit from Aunt Flo won't even make them blink.

 **TIP**: Period undies and pads are your go-to for hospital periods. Your medical crew can help you get them on and off. If you prefer tampons, that's cool, but think about what state you'll be in after surgery and if you can manage to get your tampon in and out when you need to.

PREGNANCY

Imagine your medical team as the scriptwriters and directors crafting the perfect scene for your surgery's success. Letting them know you may be preggers is like giving them a heads-up about a potential surprise guest star—a tiny human in the making!

Whether you're keeping the oven warm for a bun or you suspect there might be a bun on the way, spill the beans (or buns) to your medical dream team. Different parts of the surgery process (e.g., aesthetic) and the surgery itself might impact the baby. So, bring out the pregnancy plot twist early, so your medical team can work with you both.

Pelvis

When you're prepping for major surgery, your pelvic playground might experience a few ripples. Sometimes, surgeries can indirectly impact our pelvis, causing changes in our movement patterns or even affecting our pelvic floor muscles. Your medical village works together to ensure your pelvis stays in the groove.

After surgery, you might notice some adjustments in how you move. Your pelvic floor muscles might need a little extra love during your recovery. So, stay attuned to your body's signals, and if you ever feel like your pelvis needs some extra attention, don't hesitate to bring it up with your medical team.

Boobs

Your girls (boobs) might need a bit of extra TLC, and that's where the surgery bra comes in. Post-surgery bras are like a spa day for your chest, designed to provide comfort, compression, and just the right amount of "you got this" vibes.

Some surgeries can make our boobs play a game of musical chairs, and that's completely okay! Your left might want to check out the right side of things, and vice versa. It's like a little adventure for them.

They'll usually find their way back to each other and settle into their cozy spots. But if you're feeling a bit puzzled by their newfound exploration or if they're playing a little too much hide-and-seek, don't hesitate to chat with your Village.

"This happened to me twice. It would be mildly disturbing if it wasn't so funny. They always settled back down after having a little adventure. I never thought of post-surgery bras for open heart surgery, so I used oversized sports bras. If I had my time again, I'd get the post-surgery bras."

Urinary Catheters

Urinary Catheters are like having a temporary travel buddy for your bladder while your body heals. Sure, it might seem a bit unusual, but think of it as a pit stop on the road to recovery.

If you're wondering, "Why me?" Well, many surgeries require it, and your medical team is all about making sure everything's okay.

Don't hesitate to speak up if you find it uncomfortable or have any questions. So, strut your catheter like the temporary accessory it is!

 **TIP**: Do some hedge trimming before your surgery. Otherwise, they will give you a Brazilian haircut downstairs themselves.

"This tip is in here because when I was 21, I had no idea about the catheter. I mean, why would they be messing about downstairs for chest surgery? Anyway, I didn't do any hedge trimming; they did it for me. I was so embarrassed. I had it all sorted for my next surgery."

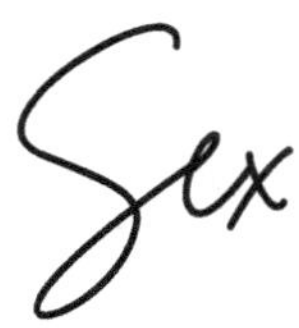

If you're curious about how surgery could impact your sex drive, or you're wondering if your libido might shift, don't hesitate – ask those questions! Your medical team has seen it all and is here to support you in every aspect of your journey.

Post-surgery, your pleasure map might take a detour, but with a little exploration and open dialogue, you'll be back to creating fireworks in the bedroom in no time!

Have an open and honest conversation with your partner. Share your feelings, concerns, and needs so you're on the same page. Your partner cares about you and wants to support you through this journey. Take a moment to chat and keep the lines of communication open.

Hormones

Surgery can sometimes cause your hormones to dance the cha-cha with your mood swings, and that's perfectly normal. You might find yourself having a full-on tear-fest during a cute cat video or laughing like a hyena at a dad joke.

Your hormones might be feeling a bit dramatic post-surgery, but hey, who can blame them? They're just trying to find their groove again. If they worry you, have a chat with your Village.

Menopause

The ultimate tag team: surgery and the marvels of perimenopause or menopause! It's like a double feature where your body decides to showcase its talents all at once. If you're juggling hormone replacement therapy or medications, make sure to sync up with your medical team. Check for any potential interactions with surgery-related drugs, and don't hesitate to raise the curtain on your concerns.

01 Stay Cool

Invest in cooling mist sprays or fans to handle those fiery moments with grace.

02 Comfort First

Keep a stash of comfortable clothing on hand for quick changes when needed.

03 Creative Outlets

Harness the power of mood swings by channelling that energy into creative outlets or meditative practices.

04 Listen to your Body

Stay attuned to your body's signals. Tune in to what it's telling you and make adjustments accordingly.

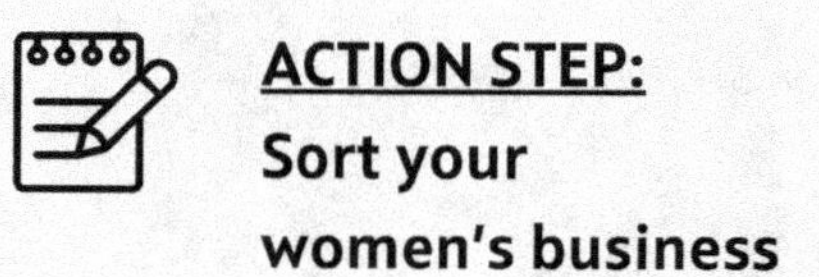

ACTION STEP:
Sort your women's business

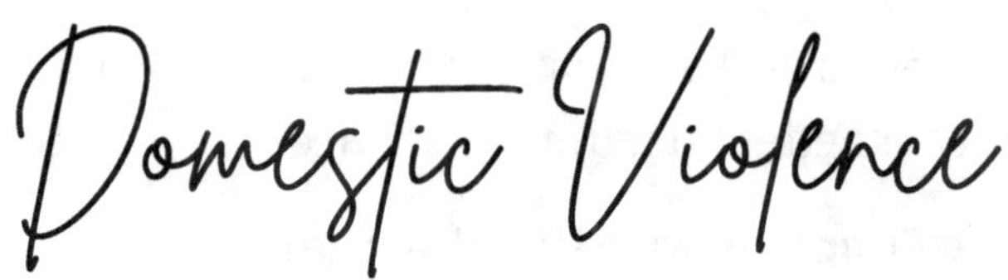

Domestic Violence

If you're facing the double challenge of major surgery and concerns about domestic violence, know that you're not alone.

Undergoing surgery can leave you feeling vulnerable, and if you're already in a vulnerable situation, it can be even more daunting.

Your safety and well-being are top priorities! If you're concerned about domestic violence, it's crucial to reach out for help. Surgery might make you feel particularly vulnerable, but remember that seeking assistance is a sign of strength, not weakness.

If you find yourself in this situation, call **1800RESPECT (1800 737 732).** They offer support and advice, and they're available 24/7.

If you're in immediate danger, don't hesitate to **call 000** for emergency assistance.

5 STRATEGIES TO KEEP SAFE

01   **Prioritise Safety in Recovery**

Plan for a safe recovery by seeking respite care or a secure

01 environment where you can heal without fear. Reach out to local shelters or support services for assistance.

02 **Share Concerns with Hospital Staff**

Tell the hospital staff about your worries before surgery or when you're on the ward. They can provide guidance and ensure your safety during your hospital stay.

03 **Build a Strong Support Network**

Connect with friends, family, or support groups who can provide emotional and practical help. A strong network can offer security and prevent isolation.

04 **Create an Emergency Plan**

Develop a clear emergency plan with steps to take if you feel unsafe. Share this plan with a trusted person who can assist if needed.

05 **Document and Protect**

Safely document any incidents or interactions related to domestic violence. Secure your personal information, including medical records, to maintain your privacy and protect yourself.

Facing surgery and domestic violence are both incredibly tough situations, but you're not alone in this journey.

Reach out for support – your safety and well-being are worth it.

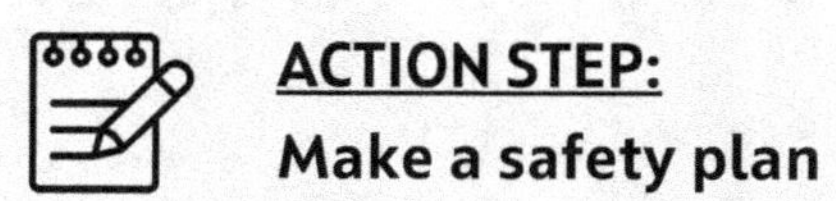

You've Got This

As we conclude this section, remember that your journey is uniquely yours, whether you're dancing with the rhythms of hormones, preparing for unexpected changes, or ensuring your safety. Embrace the power within you and let the knowledge you've gained here be your guiding light.

You're not alone in this; a community of incredible women stands by your side, ready to uplift and empower you. So, as you move forward on your path of surgery and healing, know that you are a remarkable force, and the legacy of strength you create will inspire others on their journeys as well.

"You've got this. Own it!"

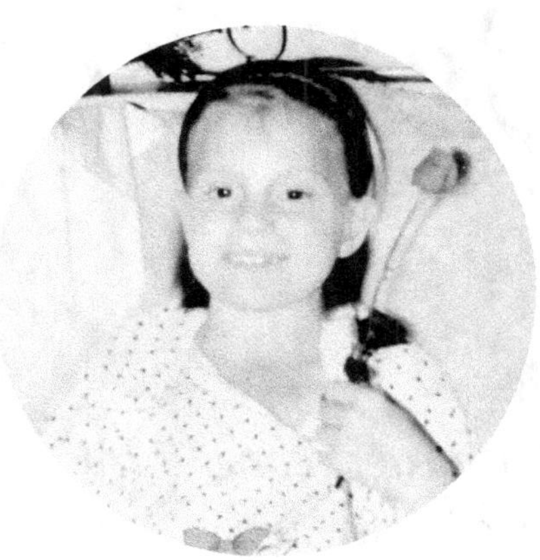

**1989 - 6 Years Old - 5 Days After My
Second Open Heart Surgery**

Men's Business

*"Major surgery can interrupt your
reproductive health and sex drive, but there
are loads of ways to manage it."*

Before we dive headfirst into "men's business," let me just set the record straight—I've done my homework! I spoke to quite a few blokes and did my research to get the best surgery tips for you.

Reproductive Health

FAMILY JEWELS

Your testicular health (aka family jewels) might not be your go-to topic at the pub, but it's worth giving a thought.

Keep an eye out for any changes in size, shape, or texture. If you're heading into surgery and they are involved, make sure to give them the VIP treatment they deserve—a comfy pillow, some cozy undies, and maybe even a pep talk (in your head, of course). So, gents, don't be shy – check your guys and give 'em the love they deserve!

DADDING

Maybe you've dreamed of becoming a dad or expanding your tribe —that's awesome! Just keep in mind that some surgeries can temporarily halt your swimmers' progress. So, if you're thinking about dadding, consider having a chat with your medical team. They can give you the scoop on how surgery might affect your fertility and offer strategies to keep your family planning goals alive and kicking.

SEX DRIVE

If you're wondering how surgery might impact your performance or if you're concerned about changes in your libido, don't be shy – ask those questions! Your medical team has seen it all, and they're here to help you score big in the game of life.

Just remember, the goalposts might shift, but with a bit of teamwork and open communication, you'll be back in the game in no time. Share your thoughts, concerns, and needs to ensure you're both on the same page.

HORMONES

Hormones can be a wild ride, influencing everything from your mood to your muscle mass. Post-surgery, your body might throw a few curveballs, like feeling more tired or hungrier than usual. Just remember, it's all part of the process, like a rollercoaster with unexpected loops.

If you notice any serious hormone-related hiccups post-surgery, don't hesitate to reach out to your medical team. They're the true hormone experts and can help you steer your hormonal ship back on course.

Urinary Catheters

Let's talk about urinary catheters–those unexpected guests at the surgery party–or, more bluntly, the tube that goes in your willy to help you pee.

Yeah, they might sound uncomfortable, but don't worry–you're not alone in feeling a tad awkward about them. It's like having a VIP pass for bathroom breaks, minus the hassle of getting up! While it might seem strange at first, it's all about keeping things flowing smoothly during your recovery.

If it's causing discomfort or any concerns, be sure to let your medical team know. And hey, don't be shy–if you have questions about this VIP experience, just ask.

You got this, and before you know it, you'll be back to your usual routines!

 **TIP**: Do some hedge trimming before your surgery. Otherwise, they will give you a Brazilian haircut downstairs themselves.

"This tip is in here because when I was 21, I had no idea about the catheter. I mean, why would they be messing about downstairs for chest surgery? Anyway, I didn't do any hedge trimming; they did it for me. I was so embarrassed. I had it all sorted for my next surgery."

Prostate

As you gear up for major surgery, it's time to give your prostate some well-deserved attention. Think of it as the captain of the pee squad, regulating your flow and ensuring things run smoothly down there. If you're experiencing any changes down there, like trouble urinating or discomfort, speak up! Don't cross your legs and hope for the best.

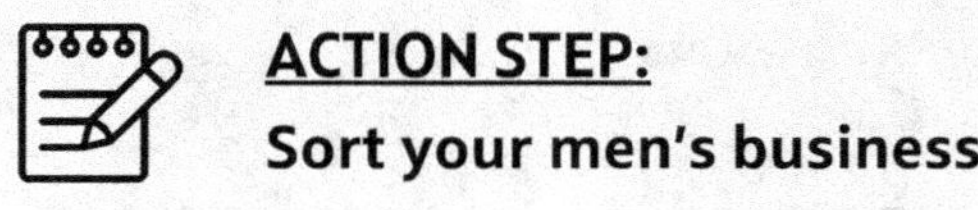
ACTION STEP:
Sort your men's business

Life Admin

"I didn't understand any of this throughout my major surgeries and wish I had of."

We're looking at the essential but often overlooked aspects of life administration, which is necessary for everyone, whether they are having major surgery or not. If the content is too confronting, you can skip to the next chapter and return when ready. I get that it's a lot to process, but this will guide you step by step.

Advanced Care Directive

An Advanced Care Directive (ACD) outlines your preferences for future medical care and your beliefs, values, and goals. It is significant because it enables you to appoint a substitute decision-maker for times when you are unable to make decisions on your own.

The value of an advance care directive comes into play when considering the uncertainties of health issues. By documenting your preferences and wishes, you provide clarity to your loved ones and medical professionals about your desired course of action in various situations.

To create an advanced care directive, you need to be at least 18 years old and be able to make decisions. The same criteria goes for your substitute decision-maker. Creating an advance care directive doesn't necessarily require legal assistance. You can include details such as appointing a substitute decision-maker, outlining your values and life goals, and expressing your preferences for medical treatments in life-threatening situations.

Give copies of your ACD to family members, your chosen substitute decision-maker, medical providers, and other relevant parties, ensuring your wishes are known and respected. You can also integrate your ACD into your My Health Record, ensuring your treating doctors can find it easily.

To create your plan, visit Advanced Care Planning:
https://www.advancecareplanning.org.au/create-your-plan

Will

Creating a will might seem like a heavy topic, but having a will in place is a profound gesture of care for your loved ones and your legacy. A will ensures that your wishes are respected, and that your assets are distributed according to your intentions.

Here are three ways to set up a Will:

01   **DIY Will Kits**

These kits offer a cost-effective way to draft your will. However, they require careful attention to detail and legal language to ensure the document's validity.

02   **Online Will Services**

Numerous online platforms provide step-by-step guidance in creating a will. They can be convenient and affordable, yet it's essential to choose a reputable and well-reviewed service.

03   **Seeking Legal Assistance**

Engaging a solicitor or lawyer experienced in drafting a will offers personalised advice and ensures legal accuracy. This option can be particularly beneficial if your financial situation is complex or requires specific legal guidance.

FUNERAL AND BURIAL

In life, there comes a moment when our journey concludes. Having clear funeral and burial instructions can provide solace to your loved ones during an emotional time. You can include your wishes in your Will. But just in case they can't dig that out fast enough, have a chat with your Power of Attorney and family.

Power of Attorney

A Power of Attorney document designates a trusted person to make decisions on your behalf if you're unable to do so due to your surgery or any other reason. It's like having a safety net that ensures your affairs are managed according to your wishes.

There are several types of Power of Attorney, including:

01   **General Power of Attorney**

This grants someone the authority to manage your financial and legal affairs for a specific period or under certain circumstances. It's particularly useful if you'll be temporarily unable to handle your life admin.

02   **Enduring Power of Attorney**

Unlike a general power, an enduring power continues even if you become incapacitated. This is a critical tool for safeguarding your interests if your ability to make decisions changes permanently.

03   **Medical Power of Attorney**

Like the Advanced Care Directive, this legal document designates someone to make healthcare decisions on your behalf if you cannot. It's focused on medical treatment and care choices.

It's about entrusting someone with your well-being and ensuring your choices are honoured even during challenging times. Consulting with legal professionals can guide you on which type of Power of Attorney best suits your situation and preferences.

Digital Age

DIGITAL ESTATE PLANNING

A digital estate plan ensures that your online presence is managed according to your wishes after you're gone. This might involve designating a trusted person to handle your social media accounts, email, and other digital assets. You might also decide whether you want certain accounts memorialised, deleted, or preserved. By leaving clear instructions, you're safeguarding your digital legacy and relieving your loved ones of potential stress in navigating the digital landscape amidst their grief.

RECORDS AND PASSWORDS

As you journey through life, you've accumulated financial accounts, assets, and responsibilities. Leaving behind a record of your financial details and passwords is just practical.

Compile a comprehensive list of bank accounts, investments, debts, insurance policies, and other financial matters. Include passwords or access information to online accounts. Share this information with a trusted family member or friend who can serve as an anchor in managing these affairs.

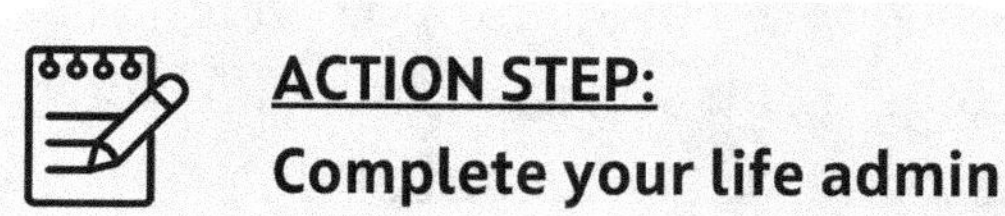

Rights & Responsibilities

"Both you and your healthcare team have rights and responsibilities. A little bit of kindness and a lot of respect go a long way in the hustle and bustle of hospitals."

Both you and the medical system have rights and responsibilities. You both need to uphold your end of the bargain.

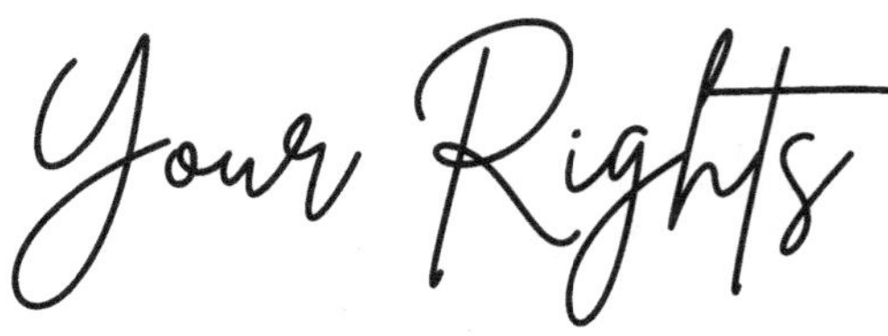

The Australian Charter of Healthcare Rights is like a set of rules that ensure you're treated well and your needs are respected during your medical journey. This is a summary of them.

YOUR RIGHTS

01 — **Respectful and Dignified Treatment**

You have the right to be treated with respect, dignity, and consideration for your cultural and personal values.

02 — **Informed Participation**

You're entitled to be informed about your diagnosis, treatment options, and potential risks. This empowers you to participate in decisions about your care actively.

03 — **Communication**

You have the right to effective communication with your healthcare providers. This means receiving clear and understandable information and having your questions addressed.

04 — **Privacy and Confidentiality**

Your personal and medical information must be kept private and confidential, ensuring your privacy is respected.

05 **Support**

You're entitled to have your family and/or support people involved in your care and decision-making if you wish.

06 **Feedback and Complaints**

You have the right to give feedback about your care and make complaints without consequences. This helps improve healthcare services.

07 **Access to Healthcare**

You should have timely access to healthcare services and, if necessary, be given information about other available options.

08 **Safety**

You're entitled to receive safe and high-quality care and to be informed about the steps taken to ensure your safety.

09 **Taking Part in Health Research**

If you're asked to participate in medical research, you have the right to be fully informed and to give your voluntary consent.

10 **Identity**

You have the right to know your healthcare providers' identity and professional status.

The full Charter can be found here: https://www.safetyandquality.gov.au/our-work/partnering-consumers/australian-charter-healthcare-rights

MENTAL HEALTH

In each region, specific laws safeguard your mental health rights and dignity. These laws ensure optimal care and support during your healthcare journey. Think of these laws as guidelines, akin to rules prioritising mental health, much like physical well-being. They outline how healthcare providers should address your mental health needs.

These laws underscore respect, your involvement in decisions, and privacy. Recognising mental well-being's significance, they deserve the same attention as other health aspects. As you navigate healthcare, these laws act as your shield, prioritising your mental health throughout treatment. Knowing these laws empowers you to advocate and decide confidently for your mental health.

Your Responsibilities

When navigating the medical system, you, as the patient, also have important responsibilities that contribute to your own well-being and help the system run smoothly.

These are a blend of various sources and may vary from hospital to hospital and State to State. Do your homework to ensure you know your hospital and State responsibilities.

Healthcare is a partnership between you and your medical team. By taking these responsibilities seriously, you contribute to a successful and positive healthcare experience for yourself and those around you.

YOUR RESPONSIBILITIES

01

Communication

It's important to communicate openly and honestly with your healthcare providers. Share information about your medical history, current symptoms, and any medications you're taking. This helps them make well-informed decisions about your care.

02

Active Participation

Take an active role in your healthcare decisions. Ask questions if you need clarification, and make sure you understand your diagnosis, treatment options, and potential risks. Being informed empowers you to make the best choices for your health.

03 Follow Instructions

Follow the instructions given by your healthcare team, including taking medications as prescribed, following dietary guidelines, and adhering to pre-and post-operative instructions. This contributes to the success of your treatment. If you have issues, let them know.

04 Respect and Courtesy

Treat healthcare providers and staff with respect and courtesy. This creates a positive and effective working relationship-essential for your overall care.

05 Punctuality

Be on time for appointments, procedures, and tests. This helps keep the medical schedule running smoothly and ensures everyone receives timely care.

06 Medical History

Keep track of your medical history, including past illnesses, surgeries, and medications. Share this information with your healthcare team to help them provide the best care possible.

07 Consent

Understand and provide informed consent for medical procedures, treatments and costs. This involves understanding the benefits, risks, and potential alternatives before agreeing to any interventions.

08 Safety

Play an active role in your safety by verifying your identity, checking medications, and confirming procedures before they take place. If something doesn't seem right, don't hesitate to speak up.

09   **Financial Responsibility**

Understand your financial responsibilities, including insurance coverage and co-payments. If you have questions about billing or costs, address them promptly.

ACTION STEP:
Understand your rights and responsibilities

Respect!

Let me make something crystal clear,

There is absolutely NO EXCUSE for abuse or disrespect in hospitals!

"I get it, pain and frustration can reach their peak, but there is no excuse to disrespect healthcare staff on the frontlines who are dedicated to your well-being. They're your partners in this journey, working tirelessly to provide the best care possible."

There is **never** an excuse to cross the line of respect. So, treat your medical heroes with the kindness and consideration they deserve. It's a two-way street, and nurturing a relationship built on mutual respect can ensure a smoother path toward wellness.

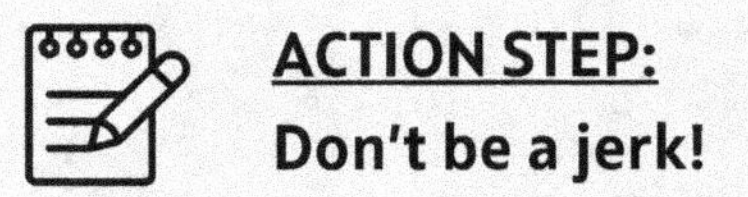

ACTION STEP:
Don't be a jerk!

Advocating for Yourself

As you face major surgery, empowering yourself involves understanding and advocating for your healthcare rights. Your journey towards better health is paved with informed decisions and active participation.

WAYS TO ADVOCATE

01

Educate Yourself

Dive into the details of the Australian Charter of Healthcare Rights to understand your entitlements. Knowledge is your armour, enabling you to voice your rights confidently.

02

Ask Questions

Don't hesitate to ask your medical team questions about your diagnosis, treatment options, and potential risks. Being curious ensures you're well-informed.

03

Clarify Information

If something isn't clear, ask for clarification. Your understanding is key to making informed decisions.

04

Seek Second Opinions

Remember, you are entitled to seek a second opinion. If you're unsure, consult another healthcare professional for a different perspective.

Involve Support People

05

Engage your family or support people in your care decisions. They can offer insights and emotional support during this journey.

Have a Notetaker

06

Having a notetaker means you can focus on your discussion and really listen to what is being said. It also means you'll have notes to keep as records.

Participate in Decisions

07

Participate actively in decisions about your treatment plan. Your preferences matter, and your input guides the course of action.

Review Consent

08

Ensure you fully understand any consent forms before signing. Read them! This is your way of agreeing to procedures or treatments; your informed consent is vital.

Communicate Preferences

09

Discuss your preferences for aftercare, pain management, and recovery with your medical team. Your comfort and well-being are paramount.

Know Your Medical History

10

Keep a record of your medical history, past surgeries, medications, and allergies. This information aids your healthcare providers in tailoring your care.

Stay Engaged

11

Remain engaged in your healthcare decisions even in moments of vulnerability. Your voice and choices drive your journey towards recovery.

Report Concerns

If you feel your rights are not respected, report your concerns to the appropriate channels. Your feedback contributes to improving healthcare services.

Remember, advocating for your healthcare rights isn't just about you – it's about fostering a culture of respectful and collaborative care that benefits everyone involved. Your journey is a partnership between you and your medical team, and your active participation ensures the best possible outcomes.

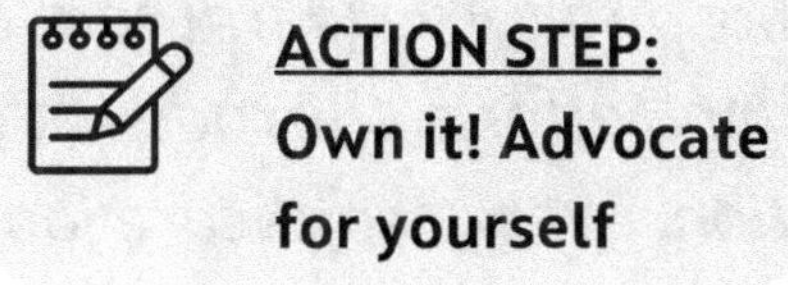

When Stuff Goes Wrong

It's important to mentally prepare for all possibilities on your journey. Life has a funny way of throwing curveballs when we least expect them, and your surgical journey might be no exception. Not everything unfolds exactly as planned, and that's okay.

"From all my four decades of experience navigating the world of hospitals, I've learnt that even with the best intentions and efforts, the road isn't always paved with perfection. Every healthcare journey has its quirks, and I've come to realise that a 100% smooth sailing isn't the norm."

Embracing the twists and turns, the little detours and hiccups are part of the adventure. While uncertainties might arise, your mindset is your secret weapon. Approach each twist in the road with the confidence that you've got what it takes to overcome it.

Take a deep breath, and let your flexibility guide you through any surgery or hospital-related hiccups that might come your way.

RISKY BUSINESS

I get it – thinking about surgery and the risks it might come with can be scary or something we'd rather just gloss over. But here's the thing: those risks are a reality that your medical team considers seriously.

You need to know the challenges you might face so you can plan for them. The best way to deal with these risks is to face them head-on. Talk to your doctors, ask questions, and share your worries. Feeling scared or overwhelmed is okay, but knowledge is your best friend here.

And remember, you're not alone on this journey – your support network is there to have your back. By staying informed and engaged, you're taking steps to make the adventure as smooth as possible.

MOUNTAINS OUT OF MOLEHILLS

Navigating the fine line between genuine concern and the usual hiccups that can happen during medical journeys can sometimes feel like a tightrope walk.

While on this adventure, trust your instincts and attune to your body's signals. Don't hesitate to raise the alarm if something feels truly off or goes beyond what you anticipated.

On the other hand, remember that not every delay or inconvenience necessarily signifies a critical issue. Patience is indeed a virtue, and sometimes, a little waiting or minor detour can be part of the journey.

Your healthcare team is there to guide you through these nuances, so maintain open communication, seek their advice, and work together to discern whether you're encountering genuine concern or simply a plot twist on your path to recovery.

RESOLVING ISSUES YOURSELF

If something goes wrong in the hospital, try to resolve it yourself or with help from your family or friends.

Start by initiating an open dialogue with your medical team. Express your concerns, ask questions, and seek clarification on any uncertainties. Your medical village is there to guide you through the maze of surgery and recovery. Don't hesitate to be the driving force behind your own healing journey.

Some practical things you can do if you feel things didn't go to plan:

01 **Communicate Freely**

If you feel something is amiss, contact your healthcare team promptly. Share your worries, no matter how small they might seem.

02 **Second Opinion**

If an issue arises, seeking a second opinion can provide valuable insights and alternative perspectives.

03 **Educate Yourself**

Understand the situation better by gathering information from reputable sources. Knowledge is empowerment.

04

Stay Positive

Keep your spirits high and approach challenges with optimism. Your mindset can play a significant role in your recovery.

05

Document Everything

Keep records of conversations, instructions, and any unusual observations. These notes can help if you need to talk about the matter later.

"At the end of the day, just remember that hospitals are busy and can be chaotic. I've had my fair share of things go wrong, but they have all been resolved easily."

COMPLAINT BODIES

If the path ahead becomes more challenging than expected, please remember that Australia has mechanisms to ensure your concerns are heard. Each state and territory has a healthcare complaints body, a neutral ground where you can voice your worries.

To go down this pathway, you can:

01

Contact the Relevant Authority

Research the healthcare complaints body in your state or territory. They have the experience and the tools to

01

address your concerns effectively.

Provide Details

02

Clearly outline your grievances and the steps you've taken so far. This will help them understand the situation comprehensively.

Be Patient

03

The resolution might take time, but your perseverance contributes to a more accountable healthcare system.

PATIENT ADVOCACY SERVICES

Patient advocacy services, often found within hospitals, bridge the gap between your concerns and effective solutions. These professionals are well-versed in medical systems, your rights, and the avenues available to ensure your concerns are addressed.

Engage Early

01

If you're facing challenges, contact patient advocacy services as soon as possible. They can help you navigate the next steps.

Share Your Concerns

02

Be open and transparent about your worries. Advocates are there to listen, understand, and help you make informed decisions.

03 **Utilise Their Knowledge**

Patient advocates are well-informed about healthcare systems and policies. Let them guide you in the right direction.

While facing bumps in the road might feel daunting, remember that you have a well-structured network to support you.

By taking proactive steps, seeking help when needed, and utilising the available resources, you're empowering yourself to navigate challenges confidently. Your surgical journey might encounter unexpected detours, but with your determination and the support of those around you, you can find your way back to smoother terrain.

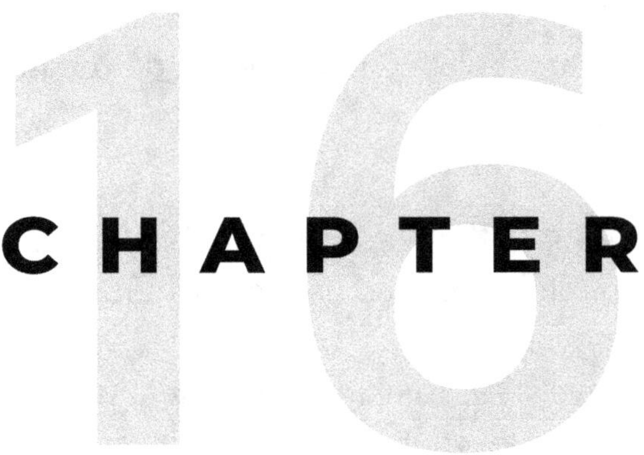

CHAPTER 16

Home Life

"There's something nice about prepping my home for my return from surgery; it's a bit like nesting."

As you prepare for your upcoming surgery, a few important things can help, like getting your home ready for your return. Your sanctuary is where your recovery takes root. Let's explore the steps that can transform your space into a healing oasis.

Prep the Kitchen

Ensure your kitchen has nourishing, easy-to-prepare meals, snacks, and beverages. You can make and freeze food beforehand. You can prep things that require minimal effort to reheat, from soups to casseroles. This pre-emptive approach ensures a rotating menu of nourishing options at your fingertips, eliminating the need for extensive cooking during recovery.

Many meal delivery services can also offer various options—from chef-prepared meals to specialised dietary choices. These services provide the convenience of enjoying restaurant-quality food without the need to venture into the kitchen.

Don't hesitate to reach out to family, friends, and neighbours who are eager to lend a hand. They can prepare meals, organise potluck gatherings, or coordinate a meal train, ensuring that you're nourished by the community's warmth and nutritious food.

 **TIP:** Pre-order groceries online and time them to arrive a day or so after you get home so you have fresh food.

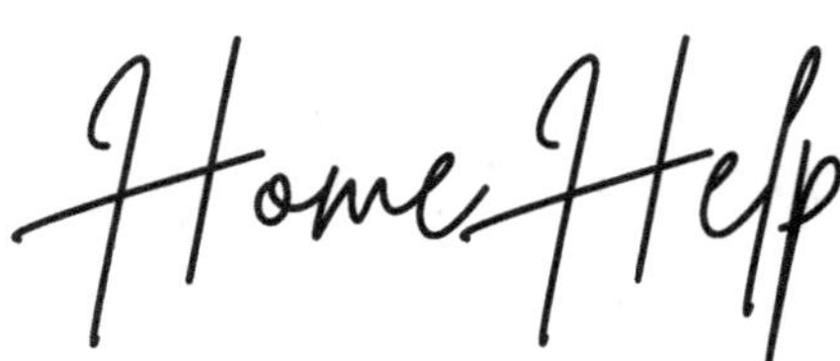

Picture a space where every necessity is within arm's reach. Prioritise setting up a designated area where everyday essentials like medications, water, and snacks are readily accessible. This strategic setup minimises the need to navigate stairs or walk long distances.

01

Restful Space

Craft a comfortable area with plush pillows, soft blankets, and a cozy chair or bed where you can retreat and rejuvenate.

02

Clear Pathways

Walk through rooms and remove obstacles, clutter, and rugs that could pose tripping hazards, allowing for effortless movement.

03

Assistance Devices

If prescribed, arrange assistive devices like crutches, walkers, or a wheelchair within easy reach to support your independence.

04

Install Grab Bars and Handrails

Add grab bars and handrails in bathrooms and hallways, seamlessly blending function with design to provide stability during recovery.

05

Bathroom Safety

Consider installing a raised toilet seat and including a shower chair or bench for safety and comfort in the bathroom.

Chores

The charm of comfort lies in the absence of chores. If you can, tackle chores before your surgery to create an environment free from added stress during your recovery. You could also consider getting a cleaner or some kind of support while you need it.

"We got an amazing cleaner at my last surgery, and he was a godsend. It meant my husband could focus on caring, cooking and tidying up, and I could focus on recovering."

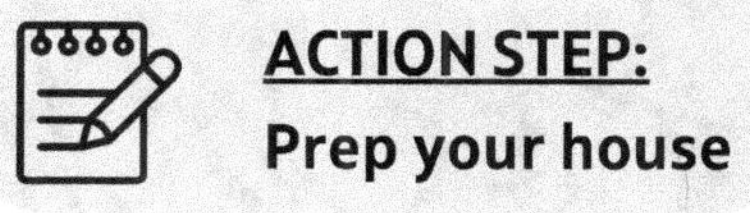

ACTION STEP:
Prep your house

CHAPTER 17

Packing for Hospital

"Making decisions before hospital makes the journey once you're in hospital smoother."

Packing for your hospital stay involves making practical decisions that ensure your comfort and well-being. Think of it as assembling a toolkit tailored to your needs.

Pre-Hospital Planning
DECISIONS

Making a few key decisions before you go to the hospital will help relieve some of the mental load when you get there. Here are a few to consider.

01 **Snap, Click, Heal**

Taking photos in a hospital sounds weird. But it can be nice to look back on post-surgery to see how far you've come and what you overcame. They can also show you what happened when you may not recall all the good things, like visitors and gifts.

02 **Accommodation**

Where will your crowd be staying while you're in the hospital? Try booking in advance for cheaper rates. If you need assistance paying for it, talk to a charity.

03 **Transport**

Think about how you're getting to and from the hospital: taxi, ride-share, public transport, plane, or your car. What's the most comfortable and convenient?

Hint: electric car seats make it much easier to get comfy.

Crown Jewels

Do you really need to take the crown jewels (jewellery) to the hospital? Probs not. Leave them at home if you can.

Pillows

If you have a really comfy pillow you love, take that with you, too. A touch of home is always nice.

"I highly recommend getting someone to take photos of you post-surgery. You might not want to look at them right away, but one day, you'll look back on them with mixed feelings. I love mine!"

 **TIP**: Take this guidebook and your Action Plan with all your notes and scribbles. They will help you through the hospital phase.

HOSPITAL EXTRAS

Here are some extra things you might like to consider for your hospital packing. They all come from my personal experience.

01 **Signs to communicate**

You could make signs beforehand for your support crew to hold up when you are intubated and can't talk. They can say things like 'water?' 'Hold my hand?' or 'Return later?'. When they are held up, you can simply reply with nods or head shakes.

02 **Nail polish**

Get rid of your nail polish. The medical team checks the colour of your nails to determine your oxygen levels and other conditions. If you have nail polish, you're stopping them from doing their job.

03 **Hedge Trimming**

If you need a urinary catheter because of your surgery, trim your pubes! Otherwise, they will.

04 **Treat yourself**

Get something new and a bit special (even second-hand). I always get new pyjamas for major hospital stays.

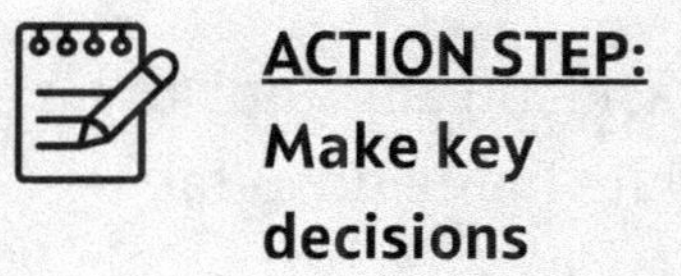

Hospital Packing List

01 **Questions**

That list of questions you've been making since you learned about the surgery. You might have run through them already, but it's good to have it if there are changes to your medical team and you have to explain again.

02 **Fashionable Comfort**

Pack those loose and comfy outfits - cozy pyjamas, roomy nightgowns, and soft robes.

03 **Toiletry Swag**

Pack a bag full of your favourite toiletries, from your trusty toothbrush and toothpaste to that oh-so-pampering hairbrush. Dry shampoo is also a lifesaver.

04 **Eyes and Ears**

Pack an eye mask and earplugs to give you that serenity now feeling while in the hospital.

05 **Medication**

Don't forget your existing meds (including vitamins).

06 **Snacks**

Pack an assortment of healthy treats and a reusable water bottle.

07 **Paperwork**

Take copies of your insurance information, emergency contact details, sign-in details, and anything else you've been asked to fill out.

08 **Cards**

Medicare, Private Health Insurance, and bank cards at a minimum.

09 **Entertainment**

Pack a mix of entertainment options - audio books, music, meditation.

10 **Chargers**

Your phone and tech gadgets.

11 **Creature Comforts**

Transform your hospital room into your comfort zone with your own pillows, heat packs, cozy blankets and anything else.

12 **Visitor Policy**

The Visitor Policy you made for yourself, including the coms plan.

13 **Women's business**

Period undies, pads and surgery bras if you need them.

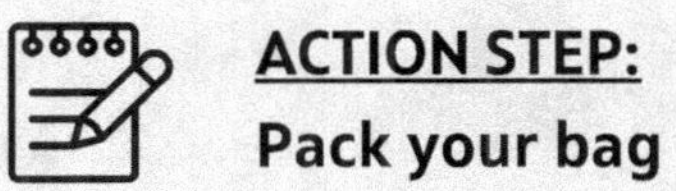

CHAPTER 18

Game Face!

"You've got this!"

Game Face

Re-read this bit when you're out the front of the hospital, ready to go in!

You've arrived at a pivotal moment, standing at the hospital doors with the deep knowledge and resilience that have brought you this far.

As you face this major surgery, remember the unbreakable spirit within you. You are ready.

The hospital staff and your loved ones have got your back. They know you can do this. I know you can do this. And, deep down, you know you can do this.

It's natural to feel nervous, but try and accept the uncertainty and dig deep. You've prepared for this; you've done the research and your mindset prep. You are ready.

Take a deep breath. And another.

You've got this!

 **TIP**: Make your own message that will resonate with you. Use it whenever you need it.

PART 3

IN HOSPITAL

CHAPTER 19

Hospital Life

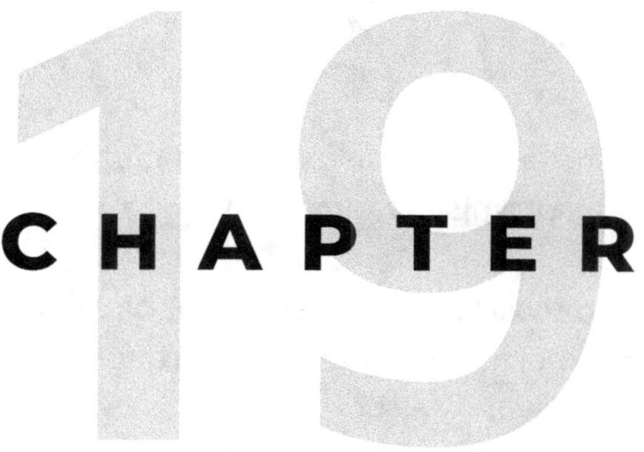

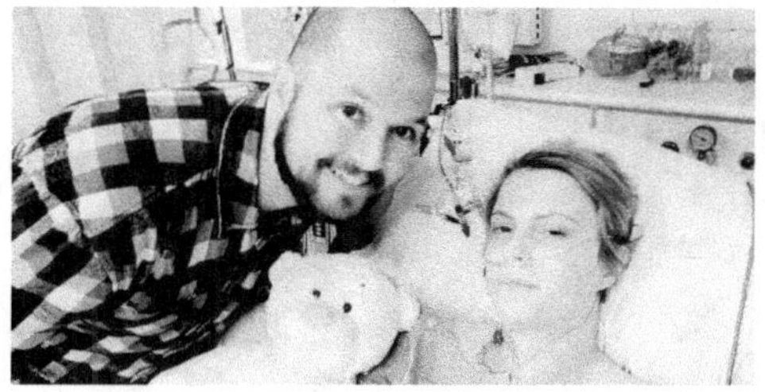

2016 – 33 Years Old – 2 Days After My Fifth Open Heart Surgery with My Husband Adam Buck

"The hospital part of major surgery really is the shortest bit, but it is the most critical."

The Night Before

The eve before surgery is a time for contemplation, where your journey meets the promise of tomorrow.

Breathe deeply, releasing any lingering doubts. Trust that the surgical team's expertise will guide you through. Feel the embrace of your support network – a chorus of love and encouragement.

Use the meditation, music or anything else you packed to help keep yourself calm.

Rest now as you close your eyes, knowing you're on the threshold of a new dawn of your life.

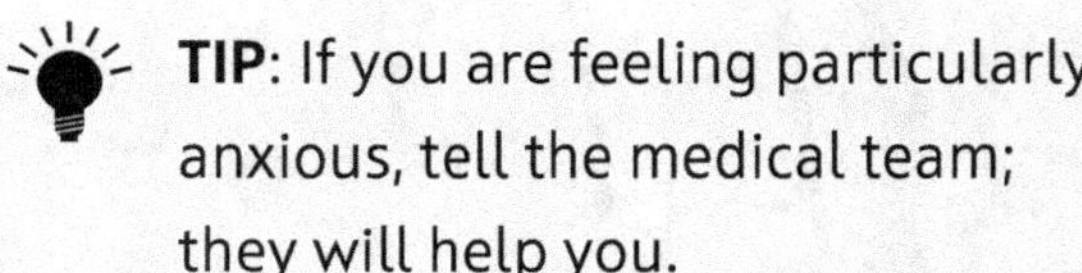

TIP: If you are feeling particularly anxious, tell the medical team; they will help you.

You've almost made it to the Game Day and you've got this!

Waking Up from Surgery

Waking up from major surgery can be a disorienting experience. You might feel groggy, sore, and confused with various sensations and noises around you. It's normal to feel a mix of relief, pain, and exhaustion as the anaesthesia wears off. Expect some discomfort, but remember that the medical team is there to manage your pain and help you recover. ASK them for help anytime!

Breathing, staying calm, and asking for assistance are crucial to coping in these first moments. Focus on small, achievable goals like drinking water, moving your fingers and toes, and communicating with your caregivers.

If you have a breathing tube, it's an unusual sensation—not painful, just uncomfortable and odd (in my experience). Removing it is pretty quick and smooth. It's also a sign that you're doing well, so celebrate it as your first big win!

 **TIP:** Use those signs to communicate with your family when you can't talk because of the breathing tube.

"I originally made these signs for my fifth open heart surgery because of previous experiences. Which included feeling disorientated and telling my family to 'piss off'. I didn't want to repeat that and needed a way to communicate when I couldn't talk. So, I designed the signs, and they worked brilliantly."

Pain Management

I want to be straight with you here – pain is a part of major surgery. But things have changed a lot since I was young. Today, dealing with pain after surgery is a top priority for your recovery.

When you're on the road to healing, remember that feeling pain is your body's way of telling you it's working on getting better. But the key thing now is to handle that pain well. It's not just about getting rid of discomfort; it's about helping you feel better overall and making good progress.

When you manage pain well, some pretty cool things happen. First, your comfort is prioritised. That means you can focus on resting, relaxing, and finding your new self. Pain can be tough on both your body and your feelings, but if you deal with it head-on, you give yourself the best chance to heal.

Also, managing pain helps you move around better and start moving early. When you keep pain under control, you're more likely to do exercises and therapy after surgery. These speed up your recovery and help you return to your daily stuff faster. Moving around also helps your blood flow and prevents issues like blood clots.

Feeling good emotionally is just as important. When you handle pain well, you reduce stress and worry. This positive approach helps you stay hopeful and confident about your recovery.

"For my last surgery, I remember laying there thinking, 'It's ok, it could be worse'. Then it dawned on me that, no, this is as bad as it gets, and I was ok. I was even thinking it could be worse! I surprised myself with how effectively I could manage the discomfort through distraction and with how damn good pain management is these days."

Your medical team is your partner in managing pain. They'll figure out what works best for you, considering your pain tolerance, history, and the kind of surgery you had. Talking openly with them is a must – tell them about your pain, what you prefer, and if you're worried about anything.

Do NOT suffer in silence!

You've also got entertainment at your fingertips now! Those devices are your new best friends. Put on your headphones and get lost in music, audiobooks, or anything you enjoy. Don't stay stuck in your hospital room – imagine yourself meditating in a forest or on a beach.

 **TIP**: Keep your device and headphones handy for anytime use. Position the hospital table so you can reach them, or press that button for help to access them.

Remember, pain might be here for a little while, but you can make it easier on your journey to getting better.

You've got this!

Perspective

You might have envisioned a more serene environment than the bustling noises and constant checks in the hospital. But take heart —you hold the power to shift your perspective and transform your space into a comforting oasis.

You've already brought your own little comforts—that cozy blanket, soothing tunes, and the trusty eye mask. These items aren't just belongings; they're the tools you've chosen to craft a sense of home within the hospital walls. Embracing them can instil familiarity and tranquillity, even with the hospital's hustle and bustle.

Let's talk about those noises. The beeps, footsteps, and chatter surrounding you are the harmonious sounds of care in action. They signify dedicated professionals tending to you and others on the healing journey. With a shift in perspective, these sounds become the symphony of healing, a reminder that you're surrounded by those here to support you. And yes, those calming playlists and guided meditations you've curated can help you create a serene atmosphere.

These simple choices help you find your balance and create an environment where healing can flourish. So, remember, within these hospital walls, you're not just a patient; you're the director of your healing story. You've brought pieces of your world with you, and by reframing the noises and embracing your comforts, you're painting your hospital stay with hues of serenity and positivity.

LITTLE VICTORIES, BIG CELEBRATIONS

Every single step you take and each little win you have are like pieces of a puzzle coming together for your significant achievement. From sitting up to doing your first poo, eating food to showering, CELEBRATE IT!

Celebrate it any way you want, with a smile to yourself, a cheer, a happy dance, whatever you want. These are the moments that matter and remind you of the strength within you. Each victory, no matter how seemingly small, is a chapter in the story of your success. You've got this!

"Celebrating every little win is important because they can pile up quickly and be motivational. Waking up is a win, getting the breathing tube out is a win, seeing family is a win, sitting up is a win, and yes, even doing a poo is a win. I celebrate every one of these things!"

Teamwork

Teamwork between you and your medical team makes the dream work. You have the knowledge of what your body is doing and feeling, and they have the expertise to get you to the end goal.

By openly expressing your needs, concerns, and preferences, you provide vital input that shapes your treatment. Simultaneously, your medical team, armed with their expertise and dedication, makes a comprehensive plan for your recovery. The teamwork between your first-hand knowledge and their medical prowess propels your healing forward.

KINDNESS

In the hospital, a sprinkle of kindness can make the whole place shine a little brighter. Sure, there might be moments when the discomfort tries to steal the spotlight or the clock ticks a bit slower than you'd like. But a smile, a kind word, or even a patient nod can work wonders. Just like a drop in a pond creates ripples, your kindness can spread positivity. The nurses, doctors, and fellow patients are all part of this shared journey.

So sprinkle kindness like confetti—in this adventure, a little warmth goes a long way!

TIP: If you want to win patient of the year take treats for the hospital staff

Physiotherapy

Post-surgery, physiotherapy becomes a vital teammate on your road to recovery. Its role has evolved from the sidelines to a central part of your care plan.

Physiotherapy is like having a dedicated coach, helping you rebuild strength, regain movement, and achieve those important milestones. These tailored exercises are your secret weapon for a quicker rebound. By partnering with your physiotherapist, you're not just bouncing back – you're propelling yourself forward.

Welcome the guidance of physiotherapy. With their expertise and your dedication, you're on track to achieving remarkable progress in your recovery journey.

"Physiotherapy changed my life! The first time I had a physiotherapist post-op was for my fifth open-heart surgery, and I've never looked back. They showed me what my body was truly capable of and how to adapt to suit my skill and energy level. I can't recommend them highly enough."

Visitors

Kick off the personal visitor policies you set up during the surgery prep. Visitors can be very comforting during your hospital stay after surgery. It's lovely to see familiar faces and share a chat or two.

If you're feeling tired or not in the mood, it's okay to put yourself first. You can say no to visitors or ask them to come back later. Your well-being comes first, and taking time for yourself is okay. Visitors are here to support you; they'll understand if you need rest. Enjoy the company when you're up for it, and don't hesitate to take care of yourself first.

"Just a note to visitors—be on time! Often, patients are watching the clock, waiting to see their favourite people on earth after what might have been a rough night. So please, don't keep them waiting in their hours of need."

Leaving Hospital Checklist

Woohoo, you made it through the hospital!! The hardest bit. Here are your questions to ask before heading home or to respite care.

01   What mediations do I need to take and when?

02   What are the medication side effects?

03   How will I know if things are not going to plan?

04   Who should I contact if I have issues (hospital, GP, Specialist, Pharmacist)?

05   What's the deal with post-surgery swelling and when will it subside?

06   What's the recommended plan for wound care and dressing changes?

07   What basic movements can and can't I do? (How do I get out of bed?)

08   When should I follow up with my primary care doctor or specialist?

09   What foods should I focus on to support my recovery?

10   What rehabilitation program will I be joining and when?

11   When can I get back to my workout routine?

12   When can I do my favourite hobbies or sports again?

13   Can I take a dip in the pool or have a bath?

14   When can I return to work?

15   When can I hit the road and drive again?

16   When can I have sex?

17   Is there anything else you think I should know to help my recovery?

ACTION STEP:
Get all your questions answered before leaving hospital

PART 4

RECOVERY

CHAPTER 20

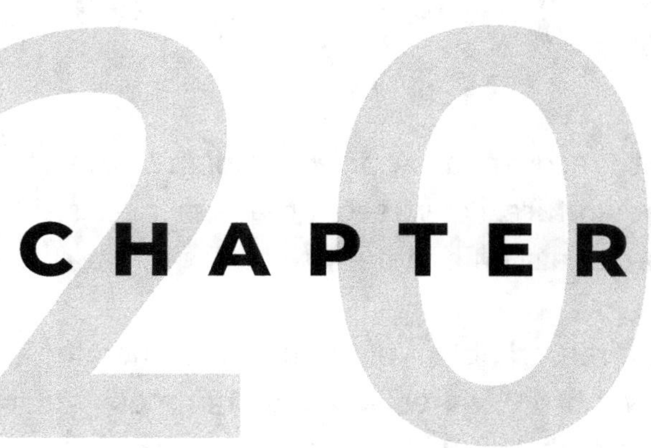

"Recovery certainly has its ups and downs, but I've always come out of it better than ever."

Road Ahead

Ah, the road to recovery after bidding adieu to the hospital is a whole new adventure. Let's keep it real – recovery isn't an express train; it's more of a scenic route with twists and turns.

Your body is a remarkable work in progress, healing at its own pace. It's okay if progress feels slow sometimes – you're building something incredible! You'll find yourself mastering new moves – from conquering that first flight of stairs to comfortably slipping into your favourite jeans. Each victory, big or small, is a badge of honour, reminding you of your resilience.

Think of this journey as an artful dance – two steps forward, one step back (sometimes). Healing is holistic, encompassing physical and emotional growth. So, while patience might not be your best buddy, it's your steadfast partner on this path. With (almost) every sunrise, you'll find yourself a little stronger, a tad more flexible, and more amazed by your tenacity.

WELCOME HOME

Welcome back to your sanctuary! The journey from hospital to home after major surgery is a milestone worth celebrating. But let's ease into this – your body is still on the mend. As you step through your front door, remember that rest is your best friend. Find a comfy spot and settle in because your body's next adventure is a recovery journey.

Hydration is essential (unless medically advised otherwise). Your body's been through a lot, and staying hydrated helps it heal faster. Embrace the art of lounging—it's okay to take things slow. This isn't the time to do everything on your to-do list—unless it's your Netflix to-watch list.

Your medications are like tiny superheroes. Keep track of your medication schedule and follow your doctor's orders like the pro you are. Let your support squad pamper you with comfort and care. If you've got any special pillows or cushions from your hospital adventure, bring them into your home routine for extra coziness. Keep resting, keep healing – you've got this!

Pain Management

When you're back home after surgery, keeping up with pain management is important.

Just like in the hospital, you've got to be mindful of how you're feeling and take the proper steps to manage any discomfort. This means staying on track with your doctor's prescribed medicines and following their instructions closely.

Alongside the medications, there are simple things you can do to ease pain at home. Gentle exercises, if prescribed by your doctor, can help your body feel better. If your doctor is okay with this, using hot or cold packs can provide soothing relief to sore spots.

Remember to listen to your body and rest when you need to. And don't hesitate to ask your support crew for help – they're there to assist you.

Staying in touch with your medical team is a big part of the game. Keep those follow-up appointments with your surgeon, GP and pharmacist. They can adjust your pain management plan if necessary and offer valuable guidance. Communication is key – let them know about any changes in your pain levels or how you're responding to treatments.

By taking an active role in your pain management, you're setting yourself up for a smoother recovery and a brighter, pain-free future.

"For my 4th surgery, I didn't manage my pain well. But, for my 5th, I absolutely aced it by staying on top of my medication cycle, using heat packs, resting, distracting myself and singing out when it wasn't working."

 **TIP**: Track your meds so you don't miss a dose or double dose. You can use an app or pen and paper. This is also helpful if you need to share your medication use with a health professional at any time.

WOUND CARE

Take special care of your post-op wounds. Follow your doctors' and hospitals' advice. If you notice anything odd about how your wounds heal, like weird colours, ooze, swelling, or anything else, get them checked out pronto!

Scar tissue is a natural part of the healing process. Keep the area clean and moisturised to help it heal and minimise its appearance. If approved by your medical team, you could try massaging the scar gently with products like silicone gel or shea butter to improve circulation and flexibility.

EMOTIONAL ROLLERCOASTER

Who knew that recovery after surgery would come with a bonus emotional rollercoaster ride? Buckle up because you're in for a journey as unpredictable as a game of musical chairs. From triumphant highs to frustrating lows, you'll be experiencing a medley of emotions. Picture yourself going from "I've got this!" to "Why is this taking so long?" in record time.

Don't worry—you're not alone. This rollercoaster tends to stick around for a few weeks or maybe a couple of months. Just like that song that gets stuck in your head, these feelings will eventually find their exit.

And remember, it's perfectly okay to feel all the feels. Go back to your mental health professional and dig into your toolkit of coping strategies. Give yourself permission to ride this wild wave and know that, with each twist and turn, you're edging closer to a triumphant finish line of emotional stability.

BODY IMAGE

After undergoing major surgery, it's natural to have mixed feelings about the changes in your body, especially when new scars or significant alterations to your appearance are involved. These changes may prompt moments of reflection and adjustment.

Remember that your body is an incredible vessel, adapting and healing in its own way. Embrace these changes as a part of your ongoing journey, a testament to your ability to overcome challenges. Talk to your mental health professional if it is worrying you.

"I've had a zipper since I was 6 (the surgery when I was a baby was on my back). So, its been there as long as I can remember. Sometimes it bothers me, but I don't know any different now, so I crack on without overthinking it."

EXCESS BAGGAGE

It's normal to have some emotions and physical responses to your major surgery experience. But, in some cases, surgery can leave people with some unexpected mental excess baggage in the form of a challenging (traumatic) experience or witnessing others on the ward suffering.

Here are some signs that you might have some excess baggage (i.e. medical trauma) and might need some help from a mental health professional.

01 **Flashbacks or intrusive thoughts**

Recurring, distressing memories or nightmares about the medical event.

02 **Anxiety or Panic Attacks**

Intense feelings of fear, apprehension, or panic are often triggered by medical-related situations.

03 **Avoidance**

Avoiding medical settings, discussions about health, or reminders of the traumatic experience.

04 **Emotional Numbness**

Feeling emotionally detached, numb, or unable to experience positive emotions.

05 **Hyperarousal**

Being easily startled, irritable, or having trouble sleeping, concentrating, or staying calm.

06 **Negative Changes in Beliefs and Feelings**

Developing negative beliefs about oneself, others, or the world, often accompanied by a sense of hopelessness.

07 **Social Isolation**

Withdrawing from friends and family or experiencing strained relationships due to the emotional toll of the surgery experience.

ACTION STEP:
Reach out to a mental health professional if you notice this happening

By sharing your feelings and experiences with a professional, you can begin the healing process and regain control over your emotional well-being. Remember, seeking help is a crucial step towards recovery, both physically and emotionally, after major surgery.

"Having 20+ surgeries and so many hospital and healthcare visits has left me with excess baggage. I've worked through it with a trauma therapist, and it has been very healing."

Teamwork

Staying connected with your medical dream team is like having a safety net of care and expertise. Your GP and Pharmacist are the co-pilots on your recovery journey, ready to answer your questions and provide guidance. Keep them in the loop – share any changes, concerns, or updates on your progress. Whether it's a quick call or a virtual chat, their insights can make a difference in fine-tuning your recovery plan.

Also, remember your follow-up appointments! Don't become lost to care, which is when patients stop attending their scheduled medical appointments and fall out of the healthcare system. This can lead to serious consequences, as regular medical supervision is crucial for managing symptoms, adjusting treatments, and monitoring overall health.

Keeping up with medical appointments ensures that any changes in your recovery are promptly addressed, allowing healthcare providers to offer the best possible care. Staying engaged with your medical team helps prevent complications, promotes better health outcomes, and ensures you have the support you need.

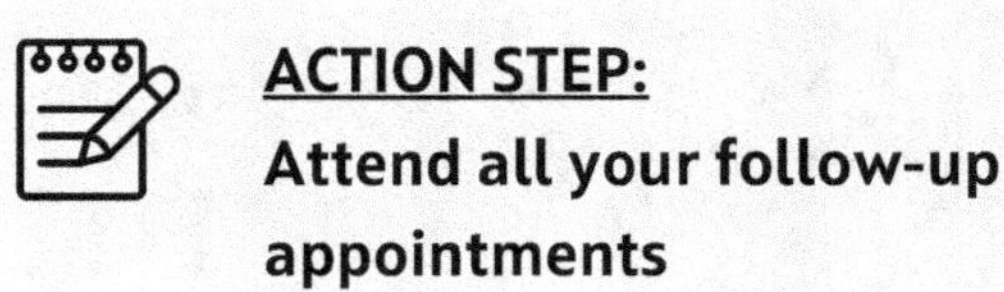

ACTION STEP:
Attend all your follow-up appointments

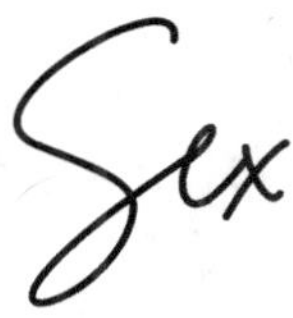

Sex

So, you've conquered the surgery mountain, and now you're eyeing another peak: post-surgery sex.

Cue the romantic music and dim the lights... or not. Let's be real – your body might have gone through some changes, and that's totally okay. It's like discovering a new dance move: it might feel a bit awkward at first, but with practice, you'll nail it (or, erm, get nailed).

Check with your medical team when your body should be ready for sex!

Have an open and honest chat with your partner—let them know what feels good and what might need a little more time. It's about both of you having a good time, so take it slow, have a sense of humor, and embrace this exciting new chapter in your journey together.

 **TIP**: If you've had open heart surgery, just be careful of your sternum. It was broken during surgery, and sex moves might need to be adjusted so you keep it healing.

Visitors

As you settle back into the comfort of your own space after surgery, welcoming visitors can be both heartwarming and overwhelming.

While having friends and family drop by is wonderful, remember that your well-being comes first. It's absolutely okay to use a visitor policy to ensure your recovery remains on track. Communicate with your visitors about when you're most comfortable receiving guests and for how long. Sometimes, a short and sweet visit can be just as meaningful as a longer one.

Ensure your visitors know that while you're happy to see them, you might also need some downtime. Your energy levels might fluctuate, and it's important to have moments of rest to aid your healing process. Feel free to let your guests know if you're tired or need a break. They'll understand and appreciate your honesty.

In today's world, being conscious of potential health risks, such as COVID-19 and other illnesses, is essential. Ensure your visitors are healthy and follow proper hygiene practices before coming over. If you're concerned about the risk of infections, don't hesitate to discuss it with your guests. Virtual visits or phone calls can also be a wonderful way to stay connected without compromising your health.

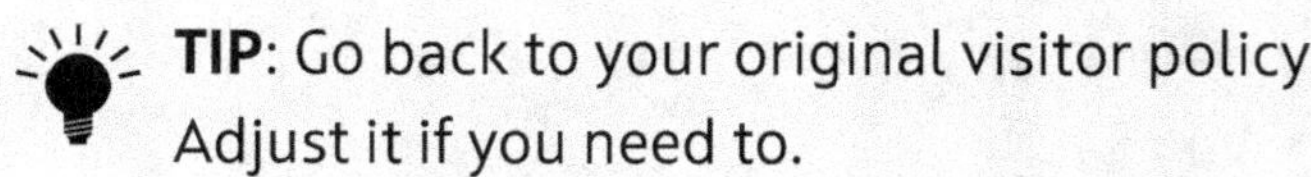 **TIP**: Go back to your original visitor policy. Adjust it if you need to.

SURGERY SQUAD

Reconnect with your surgery squad. You'll find solace in sharing your triumphs, challenges, and those "I-can't-believe-that-happened" moments. It's like reuniting with old friends who speak the same recovery language.

Together, you'll navigate the twists and turns of healing, laugh at the unexpected, and cheer each other every step of the way. Revive the camaraderie, swap stories of victory, and lean on your Surgery Squad as you conquer this new chapter of your adventure.

GET IT HERE

Facebook - Adulting Well Surgery Squad

Rehabilitation

Rehab programs are designed to help you regain strength, mobility, and overall well-being. They offer a structured roadmap that guides you through exercises, activities, and therapies to accelerate your recovery.

These programs consider your unique needs, whether you're working on your flexibility, building muscle strength, or enhancing your endurance. By being an active participant, you're investing in your body's resurgence and giving yourself the best shot at bouncing back stronger than ever.

You should be referred to a rehab program by your hospital. If you aren't referred to a rehab program, I highly encourage you to find a fully qualified exercise physiologist who can set you up with your own program. The cost of this ranges significantly. Your health insurance may cover some costs, and you can get subsidies for visits under a Medicare Chronic Illness Treatment Plan.

To find an exercise physiologist, visit the Exercise and Sport Science Australia search function: https://www.essa.org.au/Maps

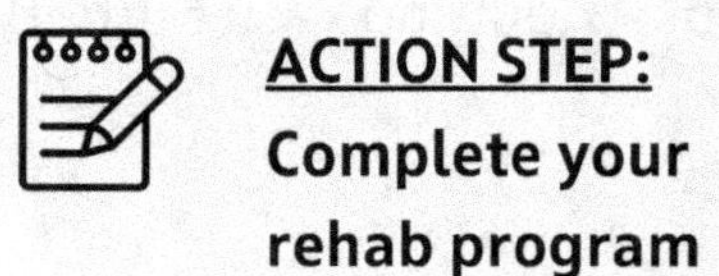

ACTION STEP:
Complete your
rehab program

JAIL BREAK

Freedom alert! But only under doctors' orders. It's time to channel your inner explorer and venture beyond the confines of your cozy cocoon. Post-surgery, it's like breaking out of captivity and stepping into a world that's been eagerly waiting for your return.

Start with small victories – a leisurely stroll around the neighbourhood, a gentle outing to your favourite café, or even a brief jaunt to the local park. The world might seem familiar and brand new, with a newfound appreciation for the sights, sounds, and fresh air.

Don't push it too hard – think leisurely promenade walk rather than an Olympic sprint. As your strength and confidence grow, so will your ability to wander farther and longer. It's all about striking the right balance between embracing the world and respecting your body's need for recovery. So, slip on your comfiest shoes, grab your shades, and let the post-surgery escapades begin!

"Rehab was the first time in my life that I learnt what my body was capable of, what pace to go at, and how to build stamina and muscle safely. It made me fit enough to walk the 14km Sydney City2Surf!"

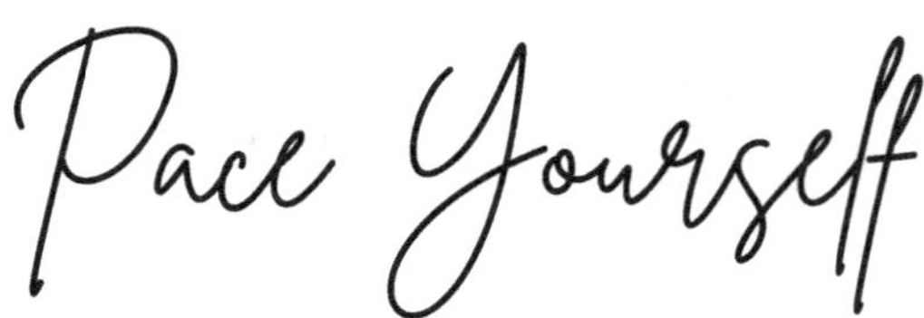

Pace Yourself

Ah, the classic recovery conundrum: feeling like a superhero with newfound energy but realising you're not quite ready for an action movie marathon. It's like your body has a memo that it's time to party, but your surgeon still whispers, "Take it easy." Grrrr!

You're bouncing off the walls, ready to conquer the world, and then... oops, you did one too many things, and you're stuffed. It's like your body's saying, "Slow down, speedy!"

You've got this, though! Embrace your newfound energy and have a secret pact with your couch. Take a page from Goldilocks and find the "just right" balance between activity and rest. Dance like no one's watching, but then nap like you're auditioning for a sleep study. It's a marathon but with comfy loungewear.

Cheers to the super annoying but oh-so-necessary part of recovery!

NORMAL, BUT BETTER

Welcome back to the rhythm of life—only this time, it's your remix! You've conquered the challenges of surgery and emerged stronger and wiser.

Now, as you step back into the familiar routines and activities that make up your world, you can redefine what "normal" means for you. Embrace the things that light you up, leave behind the unnecessary stressors, and fine-tune your priorities. This is your opportunity to build a better version of normalcy, one that's tailored to your newfound resilience.

Reconnect with your passions and hobbies, but with a renewed zest. Remember, you're not just returning to your old self – you're levelling up. As you navigate this journey back to your daily life, do it with a spark of enthusiasm and a dash of gratitude. Your comeback story isn't just about getting back to where you were; it's about soaring higher, thriving, and embracing the beauty of a life that's been reimagined.

Returning to Work

As you re-enter the world of deadlines, meetings, and tasks, it's important to do so with a blend of patience, self-care, and a dash of confidence.

You've likely already negotiated your leave and return style with your workplace. You've set the groundwork for this phase; now it's time to live it.

Flexibility is your superpower. If certain aspects of your return plan aren't quite working for you, feel free to make adjustments. After all, you know yourself best and deserve a setup that supports your well-being.

It's okay to ease back into things. Give yourself permission to take breaks when needed and communicate with your colleagues about any adjustments that might make your transition smoother. Your health and well-being come first.

Celebrate the victories, no matter how small. Finishing a project or simply making it through a full day – each accomplishment is a testament to your determination. And if there are tough days, that's okay too. Lean on your support system and allow yourself the space to recharge.

As you reintegrate into the work routine, keep your self-care rituals close. Whether taking short walks during breaks, practising mindfulness, or staying hydrated, these little acts of kindness to yourself can go a long way in ensuring a successful and fulfilling return to work.

Above all, remember that you're not just going back to work; you're returning as a stronger version of yourself, armed with a fresh perspective.

 **TIP**: If you need some extra guidance or support, don't forget to refer back to the 'work' chapter for tips on navigating the work-life-health balance like the pro you are!

 **ACTION STEP:**
Ease back into work and keep adapting as you need

Thank Your Village

As you regain your strength and are coming to the end of your recovery journey, take a moment to reflect on the incredible support system that surrounds you.

Your surgery success story was not written by you alone. It was penned by the unwavering love and care of your friends, family, loved ones, health professionals, colleagues, and countless others who stood by your side during this challenging time.

Pause for a moment and let the depth of their contributions sink in. These are the people who offered not only their time but also their unwavering emotional support. They provided the shoulders upon which you leaned during the darkest moments, the words of encouragement that acted as lifelines when hope seemed distant, and the helping hands that guided you. They undoubtedly made significant sacrifices as well to help you through your journey. They are the unsung heroes of your surgery success story.

Now is the opportune time to express your profound gratitude. Consider reaching out to these remarkable people with a heartfelt message or a simple yet sincere "thank you." Let them know just how deeply their presence has impacted your journey.

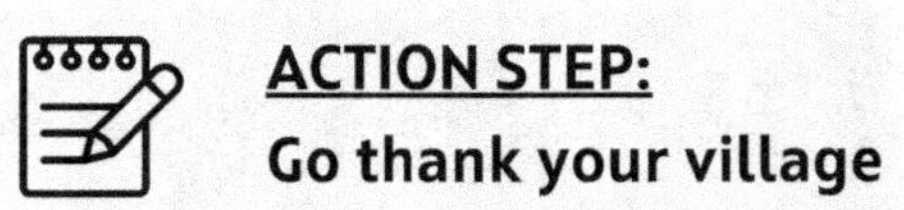 **ACTION STEP:**
Go thank your village

Pay it Forward

Having successfully navigated the challenges of surgery, you now possess a wealth of knowledge and experience that can make a significant difference in someone else's life. Consider paying it forward by becoming a mentor or volunteer for those about to undergo similar procedures.

Share your insights and tips that helped you, such as essential items to pack, the best ways to manage pain, or how to communicate effectively with healthcare professionals. Your guidance can provide comfort and confidence to others facing the daunting journey of surgery and recovery.

Another powerful way to contribute is by donating items that aided your recovery, like specialised pillows, comforting blankets, or practical gadgets that make daily tasks easier. Writing a blog or sharing your story on social media can also reach a wider audience, offering valuable advice and fostering a supportive community.

Additionally, consider connecting with a charity or hospital to offer your time or resources. Many organisations welcome volunteers who can share their experiences, provide peer support, or assist with patient education. By paying it forward, you help others and continue to heal and find purpose in your journey.

ACTION STEP:
Pay the kindness forward
and help others in need

The World's Your Oyster

Congratulations! You did it!

You've not only conquered the hurdles of major surgery but also transformed your perspective, equipped yourself with knowledge, and paved the way for a brighter future than ever.

As you close this book, remember that this isn't just the end – it's a new beginning. You've levelled up in the game of life, unlocking resilience, courage, and a newfound appreciation for the power within you.

The world is your oyster, and the possibilities are endless. So go forth, embrace your newfound vitality, and live your life with unapologetic passion. Celebrate each day as a triumph, relishing the small victories and savouring the moments that make your heart soar. The lessons you've learned, the resilience you've built, and the gratitude you hold will guide you on this exciting path.

With your game face on, your heart aglow, and the world at your feet, there's nothing you can't achieve.

Your journey is an inspiration, a testament to the incredible power of the human spirit.

Way to go you!

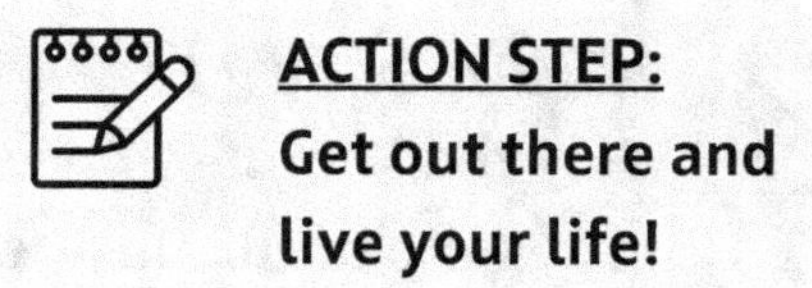

ACTION STEP:
Get out there and live your life!

PART 5

END NOTES

CHAPTER 21

Next Steps

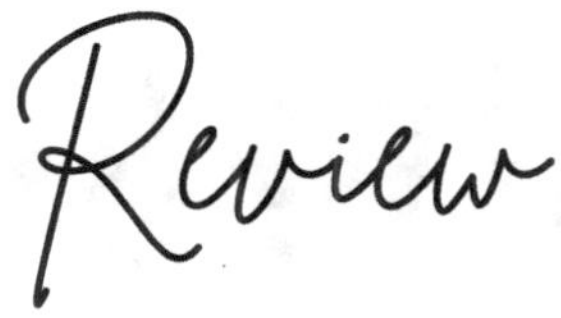

Review

I would be incredibly grateful if you could leave a review about the book! Your thoughts could be a game-changer for others walking a similar path. Your feedback isn't just a review; it's a lifeline, guiding them to a practical resource and supportive community.

By sharing your insights, you're also helping improve the book. It will be updated periodically to include your experiences and feedback.

Scan the QR code to leave a review on Google, or leave a review on Amazon where you got the book.

https://g.page/r/CSzAkXMHlLErEBM/review
Adulting Well on Google

You can also email your thoughts straight to me at
hello@adultingwell.au

Adulting Well 

At Adulting Well, we create awesome resources (like this one) so you can learn how to navigate the complexities of health, work, money, mindset and life in general with chronic illness.

If you liked this book, you'll love Adulting Well's courses, workshops, and live talks! It's everything you need to adult well with chronic illness. No more muddling through. Get the tried-and-tested methods for acing your work-health balance, managing your healthcare finances, building a mindset toolkit, and much more!

5 Star Reviews

★ ★ ★ ★ ★

"I have heard thousands of talks, and Elle's was compelling, heartfelt, and beautiful. I was really, really impressed by her story and business." - Professor Andrew Coats AO, CEO of The Heart Research Institute.

"The Adulting Well at W.O.R.K Formula can save people's lives, and it can save people's careers." - Elizabeth Boots, adulting well with chronic illness.

Thank You

"As we reach the end of this book, I want to express my deepest gratitude for taking this journey with me. Your strength and resilience are truly remarkable. I extend my heartfelt wishes as you prepare for surgery. May your procedure be a resounding success, your recovery swift, and your future filled with boundless health and happiness. Remember, you're not alone; we're here to support you every step of the way. Here's to your bright and healthy future. Take care and stay well."

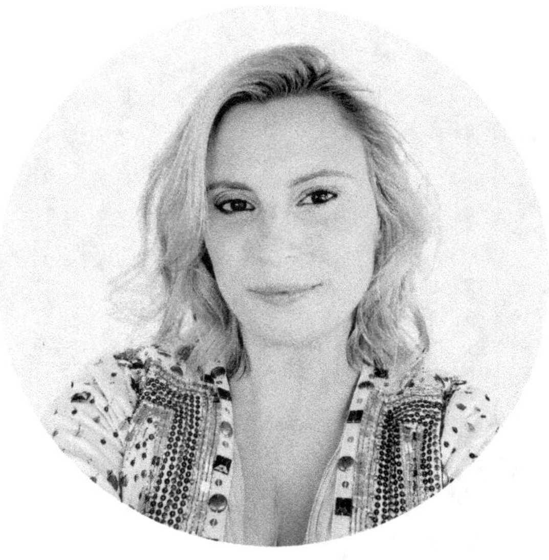

Notes